HEALING
HOMEOPATHIC
REMEDIES

A System of Healing that Works
with Your Body and Mind
to Restore Health and Well-Being

REAL RELIEF FROM THE COMMON COLD...
AN END TO ALLERGY SUFFERING...
GENTLE CALMING WITHOUT TRANQUILIZERS...
A BOOST FOR YOUR IMMUNE SYSTEM...

A LYNN SONBERG BOOK

NANCY BRUNING AND COREY WEINSTEIN, M.D.

Dell

ISBN 0-440-22156-0

US $5.99 / $7.99 CAN

9 780440 221562

50599

HOMEOPATHY IS HEALTH CARE THAT
LISTENS TO YOUR BODY,
GENTLY ASSISTS IN ITS RECOVERY, AND
HELPS KEEP YOU WELL.
DISCOVER . . .

ARNICA MONTANA (WOLFSBANE)—made from a perennial herb, it promotes healing for bruises, black eyes, sprains and strains, and fractures. If you have a physical injury, this remedy works especially well with conventional medicine.

BRYONIA ALBA (WILD HOPS)—from a vine that grows wild in England and Europe, it is used to treat headaches, fever, flu, dry coughs, laryngitis, respiratory and digestive problems.

CALENDULA (MARIGOLD)—a homeopathic remedy made from the juice of the leaves, blossoms, and buds of the plant. It is a good all-around remedy for skin problems, wounds, and cuts—applied externally as an ointment or as an internal remedy.

SEPIA (CUTTLEFISH)—prepared from the ink of the cuttlefish, this remedy is often prescribed for symptoms relating to menstrual disorders and menopause, for hemorrhoids, constipation, sinus infections, and headaches. People needing sepia are often pale and sallow, have circles under their eyes, and are chilly and sensitive to cold.

SILICA—a basic mineral remedy especially helpful for people who catch cold easily, lack stamina, or are easily worn out.

AND DOZENS MORE SAFE, PROVEN
HOMEOPATHIC REMEDIES

HEALING HOMEOPATHIC REMEDIES

Nancy Bruning
and
Corey Weinstein, M.D.

A LYNN SONBERG BOOK

Published by
Dell Publishing
a division of
Bantam Doubleday Dell Publishing Group, Inc.
1540 Broadway
New York, New York 10036

Research about homeopathic medicine is ongoing and
subject to interpretation. Although every effort has been
made to include the most up-to-date and accurate
information in this book, there can be no guarantee that
what we know about this complex subject won't change
with time. The reader should bear in mind that this book
should not be used for self-diagnosis or self-treatment and
should consult appropriate medical professionals regarding
all health issues.

ISBN: 0-440-22156-0

Published by arrangement with Lynn Sonberg Book Services,
260 West 72 Street, Suite 6-C, New York, N.Y. 10023

Printed in the United States of America
Published simultaneously in Canada

January 1996

10   9   8   7   6   5   4

OPM

The authors would like to acknowledge all of the great pioneers and teachers of homeopathy, and especially the long and strong tradition of lay homeopathy that has kept this gentle and effective approach to health alive in the United States for the last two hundred years.

CONTENTS

PART II: The A-TO-Z GUIDE TO COMMON CONDITIONS AND THEIR HOMEOPATHIC TREATMENT

PART III: A GLOSSARY OF HOMEOPATHIC REMEDIES

FOREWORD

by Corey Weinstein, M.D.

I began to study homeopathy because of love.

In 1970 I had just finished my internship at the local county hospital, where I had helped organize a free medical clinic for poor people in the neighborhood.

One of the most important supporters of the clinic was seventy-two-year-old Josephina Torres. Mrs. Torres was like a grandmother to the clinic. She brought over platters of enchiladas and chili rellenos to feed us. Her smiling face, quick wit, and encouraging advice helped enliven and inform the staff. I adopted Mrs. Torres as the kind, loving grandmother I'd never had. I also became her doctor—she was being treated daily with standard medications for high blood pressure and mild diabetes.

One day while carrying some heavy bags out to her car, she fell off the sidewalk and injured her ankle. The pain and swelling were so profound, we took her to the emergency room immediately. While no fracture was found on X-ray, Mrs. Torres had suffered a severe sprain. I wrapped her ankle securely and prescribed the routine medication given for such trouble in the early 1970s, aspirin with codeine.

While walking home from the clinic that evening I suddenly thought: *What have I done to my Latina grandma? Inflammation is the key to any structural healing, but aspirin is an antiinflammatory drug that will slow down her healing process. And codeine will decrease her awareness of the ankle pain, which is her body's way of stopping her from walking on it.*

I knew Mrs. Torres would start using her ankle as soon as possible. She would express her gratitude for the care I had rendered by standing in the kitchen cooking up a delicious platter of my favorite tamales. And I knew that her healing ability was slowed anyway due to her diabetes. It seemed to me I had made everything worse.

I asked myself: *Hasn't humankind come up with anything better than aspirin with codeine for the treatment of severe sprains?* That simple question provoked by my love for Mrs. Torres initiated a sincere and studious inquiry into the variety of health practices used throughout the world. I read about herbalism, naturopathy, chiropractic, chinese medicine and acupuncture, ayurveda, faith healing, homeopathy, therapeutic touch, massage, et cetera. I was skeptical of some and found others incompatible with my nonphilosophical mind of those days.

For someone schooled in the Western scientific tradition as I was, homeopathy seemed the most reasonable and accessible alternative. I decided to study this interesting medicinal system for a few years, and hoped I would find a way to use it in my practice. I soon joined a homeopathic study group, and met with them regularly for the next eight years.

But my practice of homeopathy did not begin in the free clinic. Friends and family were my first patients, as I learned to use the remedies for simple problems like injuries, colds, and flus. With each success my enthusiasm grew. Slowly I began to realize that I was not only studying new medicines, I was learning a new approach to health and disease. I was learning natural healing. My life and world view would be altered forever.

I learned that symptoms are the sign of the body's attempt to cope with our internal imbalances or external stresses and strains. Therefore symptoms are health functional and should not be suppressed if at all possible. The role of natural medicine is to help us use our symptoms more effectively as healing tools. Thus, the focus in natural medicine is on rest, nutrition, and gentle medicine like homeopathy. But the most profound lesson was that all illness has deep meaning to the individual sufferer. The timing and exact manner of our sickness speaks volumes about our personal strengths and weaknesses, and how we cope with the bumps in life's road. Every day I try to teach each person I see in the office these lessons so that their suffering can be used more effectively for growth, change, and preparation for the inevitable: death. In this view sickness is simply part of our creative expression as human beings, at once a mystery and a gift that speaks of our genetic history, learned behaviors, and physical-social environment. To better understand our illness is to better understand ourselves.

It is through love that I was able to break through the narrow vision I had learned in medical school. It is with that same love I present this book to you, the reader who seeks safe and gentle treatment for your troubles.

INTRODUCTION

Homeopathy is a two-hundred-year-old medical system that is used the world over and is part of the dramatic revolution in American health care. This form of natural medicine is based on the rather startling idea that you can cure a disease or ailment by treating it with infinitesimal doses of the very substance that, in larger doses, would actually cause symptoms of the disease. Homeopathy holds that *symptoms represent the body's best efforts to heal itself,* and therefore they *should not be suppressed.* Unlike conventional drugs, homeopathic remedies stimulate our own innate powers to heal ourselves—without adding any harmful side effects.

Sounds wonderful, but, you may ask: what can homeopathy really do for me and my family? Is all homeopathy the same? How will it fit in with the medical care I've been receiving? Can I treat myself and my family at home? This book will answer all these questions, and more. First, let's take a look at what makes homeopathy so appealing.

Most people turn to homeopathy simply because it

"feels right." Although they believe that conventional medicine may still have its place, their unquestioning love affair with it is over and it is becoming obvious that the high-tech approach is not effective or needed for most complaints and ailments.

Homeopathy is much more effective and gentle for stubborn chronic illnesses. Such deep-seated, long-lasting conditions respond best if treated by an experienced homeopath. If you decide to be cared for by a professional homeopath, you can look forward to successful treatment of a wide variety of frustrating conditions such as frequent infections, allergies, gynecological problems, chronic pain, psychological problems, digestive illnesses, and skin conditions, to name a few.

Homeopathy has a long tradition of self-care because it is well suited and effective for treating minor acute illnesses too. Although short-term conditions may be treated professionally, homeopathy encourages self-reliance because it lends itself to home care for a wide range of injuries and complaints from cuts and bruises to headaches, and from flus and colds to warts.

Homeopathy is for you if you want to be treated as an individual and a whole person, not just a disease or a couple of symptoms; if you want to spend more time with a health-care professional than assembly-line conventional medical care offers; and if you are fed up with treatments and drugs with dangerous side effects that suppress rather than cure. Homeopathic medicines are safer than mainstream medicines and even safer than herbal medicine; used correctly they have virtually no adverse effects, whether in the hands of a professional or used by a knowledgeable person for self-care. In addition, homeopathy teaches us about health and illness and how our physical, emotional, and mental symp-

toms interact and what they mean. It gives us knowledge and power so we can have more control over our
health and take better care of ourselves, rather than
handing ourselves over to the "experts." If you believe
the bodymind's internal wisdom and ability to maintain
and restore health should be central to good health
care, not peripheral, then homeopathy is for you.

What's more, homeopathy is an ecologically responsible approach on several levels. It uses infinitesimal
doses of medicine, so it conserves rather than depletes
natural resources, and does not create the pollution
that is the by-product of allopathic drugs. (For example, one duck supplies a major homeopathic pharmaceutical company with all the animal products it needs
to manufacture an entire year's supply of a homeopathic flu medicine.) Furthermore, because homeopathy
is a natural health-care system, it is a logical alternative
for those of us who have decided our bodies do not
make suitable toxic dumps and have cut down or elimi-
nated foods containing pesticides and additives, and
coffee, tobacco, and alcohol.

Homeopathy is for you if you've grown wary of a
medical approach that has no unifying theory connect-
ing all aspects of a disease, and is based on fragmented,
abstract, ever-shifting theories and treatments that
change along with the theories. Homeopathy is an em-
pirical science based on actual observation and hands-
on experience treating people, with a unifying theory
that explains the disease process. As conventional disease theories continue to be discarded, homeopathic
theory becomes stronger, not weaker. Scientists are
growing closer to understanding how the universe oper-
ates, and homeopathy is more consistent with this
evolving scientific theory than other forms of medicine.

On a practical note, using homeopathic care will probably end up saving you money. The medicines themselves cost less than allopathic drugs on a per-dose basis. In addition, you generally require fewer doses because they can work so quickly and stimulate your own innate powers to do the job. Because self-care is so easy and effective for many ailments, you needn't run to the doctor for every little thing, thus saving in office-visit fees. Homeopathic doctors' fees in general are comparable to those of allopathic doctors, but the homeopath spends much more time with each patient during the initial and follow-up visits, so you get more for your money. In addition, invasive diagnostic technology is used less frequently because the treatment often relieves the problem before high-tech intervention is required. Finally, treatment by a professional homeopath offers the possibility of permanently curing the underlying disease, further cutting down on visits, reducing the likelihood of long-term or even lifetime drug therapy, and preventing new disease symptoms from developing later on.

In spite of homeopathy's impressive abilities and benefits, it's important that you realize there are limits to what it can do. In emergency situations such as major traumatic injuries, "heroic" conventional medicine techniques offer the best chance of survival. And sometimes a disease has progressed to the point where there is so much destruction of organs and tissues that surgery or other conventional treatment is required. However, even in such cases, homeopathy can usually play a beneficial complementary role.

Other cases where homeopathy alone does not suffice include chronic exposure to toxic substances (such

HOMEOPATHY AROUND THE WORLD

30 percent of French people use homeopathic medicines.

32 percent of French family M.D.'s use homeopathy; 10 percent of these are using homeopathy exclusively.

100 percent of French university schools of pharmacy teach homeopathy, as do ten university schools of medicine.

42–48 percent of conventional M.D.'s in England refer patients to homeopathic physicians.

In England, patient visits to homeopathic practitioners are increasing by 39 percent each year.

In India, there are over a hundred thousand prescribers of homeopathic medicines.

The number-one-selling over-the-counter flu medicine in France is a homeopathic remedy called Oscillococcinum.

Almost all French pharmacies dispense homeopathic medicines and homeopathy is covered by state social security.

According to the FDA (U.S.), sales of homeopathic medicines recently increased by 1,000 percent.

as on the job), or poor health habits, such as eating a vitamin- and mineral-deficient diet. Homeopathy can strengthen the constitution to better withstand toxic exposure and restore health after exposure ceases, but improvement really rests on removing the toxic substance. And no amount of homeopathic medication can make up for a nutrient-deficient diet.

Still, the benefits of homeopathy far outweigh its limitations, and it's no wonder that in many countries this "unconventional" method of healing is downright commonplace. For instance, nearly one third of families in France and 20 percent in Germany use homeopathic remedies. A whopping 42 percent of British M.D.'s refer their patients to homeopath physicians. In the U.S., homeopathy used to be popular as well, and an increasing number of American medical doctors are "converting" to homeopathy as they grow disillusioned with conventional medicine. One of the authors of this book, Dr. Corey Weinstein, is one of them, and he relates his personal experience in the foreword.

Healing Homeopathic Remedies offers you information about how to treat yourself and your family with safe, natural, effective, and inexpensive homeopathic remedies. Part One contains chapters that give you a clearer understanding of homeopathy, creating a firm foundation for successful self-care. Chapter 1, "The Philosophy and Theory of Homeopathy," walks you through the fascinating principles of homeopathy and tells how it was founded by a German physician out of frustration and disgust with the kind of medicine his contemporaries were practicing. Chapter 2, "How Homeopathic Remedies Work," explains how homeopathic remedies are prepared and how they help the body heal itself. In Chapter 3, "Homeopathic Self-Care," you'll learn the basics of taking care of yourself and others—how to evaluate the symptoms, make a diagnosis, and select and administer the correct remedy.

Chapter 4: "Seeing a Professional Homeopath," lets you know what to expect if you decide to undergo professional homeopathic treatment, and includes advice on finding a qualified homeopath.

Part Two consists of an A-to-Z listing of the most common conditions—such as colds, headaches, flu, allergies, vaginitis, insomnia, and anxiety and fear—and the most often prescribed remedies for each. Also included are general homeopathic home-care measures, and advice on when to consult your homeopathic or medical doctor.

Part Three is a glossary of the most commonly used homeopathic remedies. It provides you with additional information about each remedy so that, using it in conjunction with Part Two, you are better able to prescribe the correct one. You'll be able to find most of the remedies in your neighborhood health-food store or pharmacy: mail-order sources are also listed at the back of the book, as are sources for additional information and other homeopathic products and services.

Along with other natural forms of medicine, such as nutritional therapy, homeopathy is enjoying greater acceptance in this country. In the process, it may be changing our fundamental view of how the body and mind work, as well as our definition of health. When used wisely either in the home or under a professional homeopath's guidance, this safe, effective form of health care may also change your life.

HEALING
HOMEOPATHIC
REMEDIES

PART I

. . . .

Understanding Homeopathy

ONE

. . . .

The Philosophy and Theory
of Homeopathy

Although modern conventional medicine does have its success stories, today we are seeing a growing frustration and disenchantment with the way medicine is being practiced. Our medical care is fragmented, impersonal, and growing more expensive by the minute. We use "heroic" measures: surgical removal of tumors and defective organs, organ transplants, radiation, drugs with undesirable side effects that are treated with yet more drugs, intensive-care units and "life"-support machines that seem more like "death"-support devices. Conventional medicine's main claim to fame—reduced deaths from epidemics and infectious diseases—in fact owes a great deal to improved sanitation, food storage and distribution, and living conditions.

Modern conventional medicine is not very effective against the tough chronic diseases that plague modern industrialized society: cancer, heart disease, immune disorders, viral conditions, allergies and sensitivities to foods and environmental chemicals, arthritis, and mental conditions such as depression and anxiety. It can claim few cures and is at best only able to "manage" or "control" such conditions. In some cases, conventional medicine actually causes disease: we are seeing bacterial infections resistant to our best antibiotics, and over one third of hospital patients are admitted for iatrogenic (doctor-induced) conditions. On a more day-to-day level, we take drugs that suppress our symptoms rather than help the body to heal the underlying disease. We treat something as mundane as the common cold by bombarding it with cough suppressants and decongestants to get us through the first few days of the infection; then we spend the second half of the cold recuperating from the side effects of the drugs.

Homeopathy is a totally different approach to healing. As with other forms of natural medicine, it is based on the concept that our bodies possess the innate wisdom to cure ourselves of disease, and that the best medicine is one that works with the body's and the mind's natural processes.

Like Cures Like: the "Law of Similars"

The fundamental principle of homeopathy—Like cures like—is an idea that has been around for thousands of years. Hippocrates wrote about it, and all through history a variety of cultures, including the Mayan, Greek, Chinese, and Native American, used the principle of Like cures like. However, the systematic homeopathic approach to health care owes its existence to Samuel Hahnemann, a German physician. Although his philosophy and system have been expanded and refined by several others, Hahnemann established the basic set of

principles around 1800 and gave this form of medicine
its name.

The name *homeopathy* derives from the Greek words
homoion, meaning "similar," and *pathein,* meaning
"disease" or "suffering." The name and the system was
an alternative to the orthodox form of medicine practiced in Hahnemann's era, which he dubbed *allopathy,*
from the Greek word *allos,* meaning "different." The
term *allopathy* is still used by alternative-health-care
practitioners to describe the form of medicine practiced
by conventional doctors. Then, as now, allopathy was
based on the principle that a disease or symptom is best
treated by opposing the symptoms—by using a medicine or other technique to remove, relieve, or suppress
the symptoms.

The common allopathic practices of Hahnemann's
time seem barbaric to us now. They included such drastic and dangerous techniques as bloodletting, purging,
blistering, and sweating. Bloodletting, which was done
to remove "excess" blood from an individual, was particularly gruesome. These techniques, despite their
widespread acceptance, were unsuccessful and Hahnemann stopped practicing medicine out of frustration
and disgust. One day he was translating a scientific text
about cinchona, a Peruvian bark that contains quinine.
The text attributed cinchona's ability to alleviate the
fever of malaria to its bitter and astringent properties.
To Hahnemann, this made no sense, and he decided to
test the substance on himself. After several doses, he
noticed that he developed symptoms similar to those of
malaria. Was this just coincidence, he wondered, or was
this the mechanism behind its effectiveness?

Hahnemann proceeded to test many other substances
and discovered the similarities were no coincidence.

Eventually he began to treat patients by matching their symptoms with the medicines that had produced them in a healthy person. Amazingly, his theory was supported by his experience: the medicines worked! Like did cure like, and in this way homeopathy was born.

Hahnemann and his followers tested many more substances on healthy human subjects, always noting in careful detail the symptoms that the substances provoked. Hahnemann called these tests *prüfungs,* a German word meaning "tests" or "trials," and which today is translated as "provings."

Throughout the nineteenth century, homeopathy spread in Europe, partly based on its success in treating life-threatening infectious diseases. It saved countless lives during the 1813 typhoid epidemic in Europe, and the cholera epidemic of 1831 and 1832. It has continued to have a loyal and substantial following in Europe —especially England, France, and Germany—and in India, Latin America, and the former Soviet Union.

In the United States, we have a different story. Homeopathy was brought to the U.S. by Dutch and German physicians in the first quarter of the nineteenth century. One of these was Constantine Hering, who came to be known as "the father of American homeopathy." From the urban poor to the isolated rural population, to the wealthy educated city folk, homeopathy enjoyed widespread acceptance. By 1846, it had its own professional organization—the American Institute of Homeopathy, the first national medical organization in the U.S. And by 1848, Hering had founded the first homeopathic school in the country. By the early 1900s, one in five American physicians was a homeopath. In 1900, there were twenty-two homeopathic medical colleges in the country, including Boston University, the

University of Michigan, the University of Minnesota, and the Hahnemann Medical College; over a hundred homeopathic hospitals, including New York City's Metropolitan Hospital; and twenty-nine journals devoted to homeopathy. Many homes kept a supply of homeopathic remedies on hand for self-care.

However, a number of factors converged to spell the eventual demise of homeopathy in the U.S. The American Medical Association (AMA) was formed, a publicity campaign was launched that was anti–alternative medicine, and AMA members were prohibited from consulting with homeopaths. Homeopaths began to dispute among themselves and undermine homeopathy's strengths. Up-and-coming sophisticated modern technology, such as painkillers, anesthesia, antiseptic practices, and improvements in hospital care, enhanced the reputation of allopathic medicine. The state and local medical societies began to accept homeopaths, and many homeopaths were thus absorbed, gaining respectability, but effectively co-opting and weakening the homeopathic community.

By 1918, the twenty-two homeopathic colleges were down to seven and homeopathy nearly disappeared completely in the U.S. Modern orthodox medicine continued to evolve—bloodletting and other "heroic" procedures were replaced by more powerful drugs, and diagnostic surgical techniques became more sophisticated, safer, and less painful. Antibiotics seemed to produce miraculous cures more "efficiently" than homeopathic remedies, which required time-consuming individualized treatment. These developments were not limited to the U.S., but this country more than any other seemed to believe and trust in the new technology. As immigrants embraced the new, they rejected anything that smacked of being old fashioned, backward, or from "the old country"—including folk medicines such as herbalism and homeopathy.

Why Symptoms Should Not Be Suppressed

Today's allopathic medicines, which aim to counteract symptoms, are prescribed on the basis of dissimilarity. We have antihistamines for allergies, antitussives for coughs, antacids for stomach problems, antibiotics for infection . . . all of which "work" by suppressing the symptoms without treating the underlying diseases that produce the symptoms. This results in palliation (soothing) of your original symptoms, but also a dependence on the drug as well as undesirable side effects. It's easy to become addicted to allopathic drugs, from tranquilizers to stimulants, and antacids to nose drops, because of the rebound effect and because they do not cure.

Such suppression is like smashing a beeping smoke alarm instead of putting out the fire. The smoke alarm is a sign that something is wrong and needs to be attended to. Attending to the superficial warning fixes the immediate problem of annoying beeps, but will not repair the underlying problem, which will only lead to greater problems later on.

The Like-cures-like principle is not unknown in allopathic medicine, but it is enlisted only occasionally and, even then, incompletely and in comparatively crude forms. For example, certain immunizing vaccinations use small doses of allergens; digitalis, which is toxic to the heart, is used in small doses for heart failure; small amounts of colchicine, which causes symptoms of gout, are used to treat this condition; and gold, which causes joint pain, is used to treat arthritis. Cancer treatment is turning toward immunology, which seeks to stimulate and mimic the body's natural defense responses. However, these are mere nods to the Law of Similars and do not incorporate any of the other distinguishing features of homeopathy, such as individualization of treatment and extremely safe, low doses.

Homeopathic remedies, through sophisticated, subtle, and holistic applications of the Law of Similars, never aim to suppress symptoms. As we shall see later, they work on a deeper level to help the body's own healing powers correct the root causes of our health problems. Homeopathy works with, rather than against, your body, by seeing disease and symptoms in a different light.

Symptoms as Defenses

In homeopathy, your symptoms are not the enemy, not something to be fought tooth and nail. Unlike allopathic medicine, symptoms are not confused with the disease itself. They are seen as your body's best efforts to deal with a disease—your body's unique way of expressing that a disease is present and that it is mounting a defense against the disease. According to homeopathy your symptoms, therefore, may be unpleasant, but they should not be suppressed. Rather, they should be stimulated and supported so they can do their job more effectively, more efficiently, and your body can better rid itself of the disease and return to health.

An oft-cited example of our healing ability is the use

of fever. When bacteria or viruses grow out of control, your body responds by creating fever, and the higher temperature accomplishes several things. It spurs the production of an antiviral substance called "interferon"; it increases the activity of your white blood cells, which fight infections; and it slows down the activity of bacteria, making them more susceptible to attack. Homeopathy has long appreciated fever as a powerful natural healing mechanism, that your ailing body "knows" to produce.

Allopathic medicine is only beginning to realize that unless your fever is raging so high that it could cause damage, high temperature should not be lowered artificially with drugs such as aspirin or acetaminophen. This could actually prolong the course of the infection (and, in the case of aspirin, could lead to a dangerous condition called Reye's syndrome in children). Other examples include coughing, which helps clear breathing tubes and rid the body of mucus and dead pathogens; diarrhea, which speeds the evacuation of pathogens and irritants from the bowel; and vomiting, which empties the stomach of harmful or poisonous substances.

Your symptoms may not always serve such clear therapeutic purposes, but according to homeopathy, they are always evidence that your body is trying to heal itself. As such, they provide clues toward a natural pathway to health, which your body is not always strong enough to complete on its own. Although our bodies are wise and capable, they sometimes need a boost or catalyst to stimulate their natural tendencies. Homeopathic remedies provide that catalyst, in an individualized and highly systematic way, and without harmful side effects.

The Totality of Symptoms

Another key concept in homeopathy is that you do not exist solely on a physical plane—you also have a non-physical dimension including the mind and the spirit. These three—body, mind, and spirit—are inseparably intertwined. They work together to create the marvelously unique individual that is each one of us. Homeopaths refer to this as the "bodymind."

It follows that your symptoms also exist on all three planes, and that together your symptoms form a unique pattern, or a complete picture, of your illness. For example, although a headache may be your main complaint, it may also be accompanied by a particular kind of lower-back pain; you may notice you are in a particular mood, and be irritable or sad; you may feel weak and tired at two o'clock in the afternoon, a time when you are usually full of energy; and you may feel strangely forsaken at times. Allopathic doctors may take into account a collection of physical symptoms in addition to your headache—such as visual disturbances and nausea—but these only serve to pigeonhole the type of headache, such as migraine.

The complete bodymind picture is known as the "totality of symptoms" and is what a homeopath seeks to discover when he or she takes your case history. Although your symptoms are important in deciding on the appropriate treatment, the goal is not to treat your symptoms per se; rather they are a guide to match the medicine to your bodymind's underlying disease.

The goal in homeopathy is to help you restore health and balance to all three planes. Clearly, eradicating or suppressing one or two symptoms does not restore balance to your bodymind totality. Allopathic medicine is only beginning to recognize the interrelatedness of mental and physical health. For example, in clinics that specialize in treating chronic pain, physicians recognize that pain is often accompanied by an emotional state of depression and anxiety and may attempt to treat this with an antidepressant. In their view the pain produces the depression, and there is a straight line between cause (pain) and effect (depression). Homeopathy recognizes that there is not necessarily a direct cause-and-effect relationship; instead, the symptoms are components of a total web—they are connected and interact with each other in subtle and important ways.

In spite of its occasional flirtation with "holism," allopathy generally still focuses on the major physical complaint or a few physical complaints as a means of diagnosing, naming, and treating a disease. Homeopathy, however, doesn't even recognize distinct common diseases in the same way you are used to. It doesn't group all headache patients together, or cancer patients together, or heart-disease patients—and it doesn't treat them as a group either. Five people with angina each might walk out of the homeopath's office with a different medicine, depending on their total symptom picture. Homeopathy recognizes that although people may share similar symptoms—such as a solid tumor in the same organ in the case of cancer, or chest pain in the case of heart disease—there are considerable variations among people, and the treatment should reflect that variety. The changes or symptoms are the results of disease, they are not the disease itself.

Homeopaths may use certain terms to label a disease or condition that best summarizes a standard diagnostic entity, such as flu or cold, but this is generally to help you understand the diagnosis. For simplicity of communication, we have used such labels in this book as well. But your flu is not the same as your uncle Charlie's flu, even though you may share a few symptoms. In a sense, the symptoms are your own unique creation, your own way of responding to whatever is the "cause" of your illness. Every day, in sickness and in health, you write your own novel or paint your own painting—and at the same time you are the pages or the canvas.

Your Vital Force

Homeopathy proposes that we all have a vital force, or life force, that sparks and organizes our existence. It is suffused throughout our being and connects the physical, spiritual, and mental planes and keeps them healthy. This primordial organizing force may be thought of as a form of intelligent energy.

This concept encompasses your innate power to heal, and is also central to other philosophies and forms of medicine; these include traditional Chinese thought and medicine (where it is called "chi") and Indian philosophy (where it is known as "prana" or "kundalini"). In the *Star Wars* movies, it was called simply "the Force."

Part of your vital force is a natural healing effort. This has been underrecognized in allopathic medicine; but you can see it in action when a placebo (sugar pill or fake medicine) is given. A placebo is often given to one group of subjects in an experiment, while another group gets the active or "real" medicine. The researchers can then compare the results of the two and see if the real medicine has any effect. Often, there will be a beneficial effect from the "placebo" as well—in 30 percent or even 50 percent of the time.

Physicians dismiss this and trivialize it as "just the placebo effect," rather than giving this phenomenon its due respect. Instead of "placebo," we should be calling it "the self-healing effect." There are many cases of incurable diseases being cured without medical treatment, and of terminally ill people living way beyond their doctors' predictions. Such spontaneous remissions are also the healing efforts of the vital force at work. Conventional medicine cannot rationally explain this healing intelligence, which is our miraculous healing ability.

Homeopathy considers all illness to be a weakness, disturbance, or blockage of the vital force, which your body tries to correct by creating physical, mental, and emotional changes called symptoms. It is your vital force using the tools at its disposal to heal itself. Your vital force is in some ways not totally comprehensible on an intellectual level. It is partly genetically determined, but it is not material—it is ethereal. It is hard to influence, but not impossible. Yogis do it through yoga and meditation; acupuncture does it through affecting the channels through which it flows. You strengthen it on a day-to-day basis with various health habits through diet, exercise, stress management, relaxation, and sleep. And when your vital force is not up to doing the job alone, homeopathy steps in to give you a helping hand and move you along the path to wellness.

The Homeopathic View of Diseases

In homeopathy, there are essentially two types of disease or illness: acute (short-term) illness and chronic (long-term) illness.

Acute diseases. When you have an acute disease, you have symptoms that are profound—often incapacitating—and appear suddenly. Fortunately, they are also of relatively short duration. They are self-limiting, meaning that after they peak, they go away by themselves through the natural healing efforts of the vital force. Such acute diseases are rather simple and easy to treat homeopathically. Since self-care is generally safe and effective, these are generally the types of conditions you'll learn to treat in this book.

Acute illnesses can result, for example, from the arrival of an influenza epidemic, an overload of bacteria in contaminated food, an injury such as a burn or sprain, an exposure to a toxic chemical, or a saddening experience such as the death of a loved one. Since homeopathy considers symptoms to be the means by which your innate healing effort rids you of the disease, homeopathy helps by making your symptoms more effective. It accelerates the healing process so symptoms can go away more quickly, because your body doesn't need them anymore.

Homeopathy also seems to soothe acute symptoms and make them more tolerable—even if you still have symptoms, they don't bother you as much. Homeopathic medicines alleviate discomfort and palliate symptoms without suppressing them. This is in stark contrast to allopathic medicine, which makes symptoms go away by preventing your body from creating them. With aspirin, cough medicines, and decongestants, you feel better at the time, but do nothing to speed actual recovery.

Homeopaths believe such suppressive drugs drive the disease deeper and help transform it into a chronic condition. In fact, aspirin has been shown to prolong acute diseases. Homeopathic remedies also prevent the lingering effects of subacute illness (such as the nagging cough that drags on and on after a cold). It also strengthens your vital force over time rather than debilitating it, much as the immune system has been shown to gain strength after successfully battling infections.

Some of your acute reactions are not illnesses per se —they are quite superficial and are due rather to external influences such as anemia or fatigue caused by poor diet or other bad habits, or coughing caused by smoking. Homeopathic remedies are generally not called for to cure this type of condition; removing the cause is preferred.

Chronic Diseases. When you have a chronic disease, the symptoms are more persistent and can last months, years, or an entire lifetime. They are characterized by a repetitive pattern of symptoms, which may or may not be debilitating. Chronic diseases may be progressive and produce a relentless worsening of your symptoms over time, with increasing levels of disability. Or your symptoms may change with the passage of time, but your underlying disease stays the same.

Chronic diseases are more deep seated than acute diseases, and they do not generally go away with the vital force acting alone. Although a chronic disease may send up acute symptoms from time to time that then recede temporarily, you should not confuse these flare-ups with self-limiting acute diseases. Rather, they are acute crises that your bodymind creates and that signal an underlying disturbance.

Examples of chronic diseases are asthma, rheumatoid arthritis, cancer, heart disease, diabetes, drug and alcohol addiction, depression, anxiety, insomnia, multiple sclerosis, eczema, hay fever, bronchitis, and migraine headaches. Chronic disease varies in severity—your symptoms may remain mild (for example, three days of hay fever during the year); or moderate (for example, painful menstrual periods requiring medication every month); or progress to severe symptoms in which there may be lethal organ failure (heart failure or emphysema). Chronic diseases exist for a variety of reasons—because of a genetic predisposition or weakness, allergic tendencies, through infection, massive or chronic exposure to toxic substances, or unhealthy habits such as cigarette smoking.

Although chronic diseases are difficult to soothe and cure because they can be complex and are so deep rooted, homeopathy has much to offer. In most instances, chronic disease is serious and you should be treated by an experienced professional homeopath. This is particularly true if you have had the disease for years and have been taking strong allopathic medication, which would be dangerous to stop on your own, or if your disease is so severe that you have been admitted to a hospital because of it. However, if you have a mild chronic condition, or a moderate one with infrequent crises, you may find a condition in this book that matches yours, and you may find an effective homeopathic remedy. But before proceeding be sure to read the warning signs that indicate when you should see a professional.

Medicines used to cure chronic conditions are called *constitutional remedies* because they work on such a deep level. Because chronic conditions are so entrenched, they usually take a long time to cure. Homeopathic remedies correctly prescribed for chronic disease strengthen your vital force and add to its knowledge. They gradually reduce the episodes of acute flare-ups while helping your bodymind cure the underlying disturbance. As homeopathy cures, it also helps prevent future problems.

Infectious Disease: Germs and Susceptibility

Infections are nothing more than parasites living off the human organism. Many of these parasites are ubiquitous in our lives and in our bodies and normally do not cause problems until, for some reason, they grow out of control. Others are rare or new to our lives and catch us by surprise. These parasites include microorganisms ("germs") such as bacteria and viruses; fungi; one-celled creatures such as protozoa and amoeba; and worms and insects. They can invade anywhere, including your upper respiratory tract (colds); skin (ringworm, athlete's foot, lice); digestive tract (amoebic dysentery); genitourinary organs (venereal disease, vaginitis, cystitis); and immune system (HIV).

Homeopathy recognizes that the "germ theory" plays a role in determining who will succumb to infection and how severe it will be. This includes the frequency and volume of exposure: everyone is at higher risk during an epidemic or the flu season, or in a situation such as a day care center where germs are plentiful and passed easily by close and frequent contact. Another factor is the relative invasiveness and infectiveness of the parasite: some critters are simply stronger and more aggressive than others, and an organism such as a virus tends to gain strength during the course of an invasion. Simple precautions such as sanitation and proper hygiene go a long way in preventing infections from taking hold.

Homeopathy also gives great weight to the susceptibility of the "host" to its "guests." The presence of a parasite is not the sole cause of your infection; rather, it is the result of a previously established disease that leaves you more susceptible. Your susceptibility is influenced by many factors, including psychological and physical stress, nutrition, and heredity. Susceptibility explains why some people rarely get colds, flu, or other infectious diseases, even while nursing the sick; and why others "catch everything" and suffer multiple colds during the year.

Infection may be an acute, self-limiting disease that is part of normal living and serves to actually strengthen the immune system. If you suffer from multiple or recurrent infections, however, it is usually a sign of chronic disease and weakness of your vital force. In either case, homeopathy offers what allopathy cannot: a tool that both helps you throw off the infection and strengthens your constitution so you are less susceptible in the future. Homeopathy creates a less hospitable environment so the infectious agent can no longer thrive.

Allopathy, on the other hand, enlists symptom-suppressing drugs, including antibiotics and antifungals that "kill" the invading organism. This approach has gotten seemingly spectacular results, and no doubt such strong drugs can save lives when infection is severe. However, there is a price to pay in both the short and long term. Antibiotics often have troublesome side effects, and some people are highly allergic to the drugs. Antibiotics prescribed to eradicate a certain bacterium also kill friendly bacteria, such as those required to digest food and produce certain vitamins. Other bacteria, normally held in check, may thrive, causing additional infections. Overuse and misuse of antibiotics has caused resistant strains of bacteria to develop, rendering these drugs worthless for any future treatment. And antibiotics only work against bacteria—they do not work at all against viruses. Finally, allopathic antiinfection drugs do nothing to remove your susceptibility to future infection.

For all these reasons, homeopaths believe homeopathic remedies are the best way to treat infection, although most would agree that under certain conditions —very severe infections, where time is of the essence— antibiotic treatment may be best for the patient, used in conjunction with homeopathic care. But in most instances, homeopathy can speed your recovery from mild, recurrent conditions such as low-grade viral infections and vaginitis, flu, sinusitis, bronchitis, and ear infections—as well as from more serious diseases. Often homeopathic self-care is a safe and effective means of speeding recovery.

Homeopathy was far more effective than allopathy during the terrible epidemics that swept through Europe and the United States in the 1800s. The death rates in homeopathic hospitals were as little as one half to one eighth the rate in orthodox hospitals. During the cholera epidemic in Cincinnati, for example, 3 percent of homeopathically treated patients died, versus 48 to 60 percent of conventionally treated patients. Studies suggest and physicians report that homeopathy may be effective in strengthening immune systems and reducing opportunistic infections in people with HIV infection. Chapter 2 describes the major scientific studies on homeopathy, immunity, and infectious disease.

TWO

· ·

How Homeopathic Remedies Work

Homeopathy differs from other types of medicine, including the natural medicines, in the way the remedies are prepared, or potentized. There is no concrete explanation as to why this method, which involves extremely diluted substances, should produce such effective remedies. Homeopaths are unable to provide an explanation as to how Samuel Hahnemann developed this technique, or as to the mechanism by which it works. Yet homeopathic remedies have worked—sometimes dramatically—time after time for nearly two hundred years. There is a growing body of scientific evidence supporting homeopathy's effectiveness. These new findings also provide promising clues and theories that may begin to explain why homeopathic remedies work so often.

The Homeopathic Provings

Provings are the research technique by which homeopaths learn about the symptoms produced by a substance. When Hahnemann began his provings, he studied herbs and other medicinal substances used at the time. Unlike allopathic drugs, which are first tested in test tubes, then animals, and finally in sick human patients, homeopathic remedies are first tested or proved in healthy humans. Otherwise, the symptoms of the sick person could get mixed up with symptoms caused by the remedy. The only way we can obtain an accurate symptom picture is to allow the remedy to express itself in as pure a form as possible.

For each remedy, a number of "provers" (healthy test subjects) are required. The provers take a single dose of the substance; or they take several doses if necessary to elicit the toxic symptoms. Once symptoms appear, they stop taking the remedy. The prover must keep careful records of his or her reactions; and also whether the symptoms are affected by factors called "modalities": movement, eating, drinking, weather changes, the time of day, and so on. Additional information is obtained through interviews. The researchers meticulously record all the symptoms and then combine the reported symptoms of all the provers for that remedy to get as complete a picture as possible.

According to homeopathy, any substance that has a proven effect on a healthy person can potentially become a remedy. Hahnemann proved about sixty medicines in his day, and this number has since been enormously expanded. Today, over two thousand substances have been proved homeopathically; however, the average homeopath uses between two hundred and three hundred remedies on a regular basis. They consist of a wide variety of substances; most (about 80 percent) are from plants, the rest are derived from minerals and animal products (about 10 percent each). Remedies are prepared from such substances as dandelion, plantain, corn, arsenic, salt, venom from poisonous snakes, and ink from a cuttlefish, and even allopathic drugs such as penicillin (which is made from a mold). The mainstay or "bible" for homeopaths is *The Homeopathic Materia Medica,* which contains alphabetically arranged individual listings of each proven remedy with the information obtained from the provings. The symptoms listed for each remedy usually didn't appear in each one of the provers, and they usually do not appear all at once in the patients either. Some people are more sensitive and so have more symptoms, but some symptoms are highly characteristic and appear most frequently.

Homeopaths are still conducting provings today, and publish the new remedies in updated materia medica. They also appear in the various homeopathic journals, which are generally published quarterly. For example, ash from the Mount Saint Helens volcano was recently proved and the results published. Few people realize it, but in a sense, homeopathic remedies are not the only ones that have been "proved." If you take a look at the label or package insert of any conventional prescription or nonprescription drug, you'll see that in addition to the primary desired effect, there are a variety of side effects. Looking up the drug in a book such as a consumer's guide to drugs or *The Physician's Desk Reference* (available at libraries, pharmacies, and doctors' offices) will produce an even longer list for each drug. These adverse reactions or side effects could be considered to be the symptom picture that results from the unintended proving of the drug. Yet they are prescribed to a wide variety of people who share only one symptom that would be affected by the drug; all the other effects are considered to be adverse, or side effects. They may be unintended, but they are nevertheless real.

Potentization: Preparing the Remedy

At first Hahnemann conducted his provings using the relatively large doses of medicine which were customary in that era. When he subsequently applied the medicines to his sick patients, he logically used the same high dosages. This arrangement, however, appeared to aggravate the patients' symptoms before they got better. For example, if one of the symptoms was a cough, the person might experience a temporary but distressingly violent coughing fit.

Hahnemann's response was to try reducing the dose. This approach, he found, was successful: there was less aggravation of symptoms, but the person still got better. He continued to reduce the dose systematically until he reached a point where no detectable residue remained in the dilution. At some point—no one knows how—he discovered that by *succussing* (vigorously shaking or vibrating) the solution, he was able to increase or *potentize* the diluted medicine's effectiveness. He found that with each dilution and succussion of the medicine, it actually became stronger, while the likelihood of symptom aggravation was reduced. In other words, the smaller the amount of the original substance in the solution, the higher the potency.

This extreme example of *Less is more* has been very hard for nonhomeopathic scientists to accept, and is basically unheard of in allopathic medicine and traditional pharmacology, where the accepted doctrine is: The more of the drug, the bigger the effect.

Hahnemann believed that succussion somehow re-leased the remedy's curative powers. Today's ho-meopaths believe the remedies work on a deeper level than conventional drugs—one that is subtle and basi-cally nonphysical. But, most people want to know: Ex-actly how diluted are the remedies? Do they really work? And what is the likely explanation of how they work?

The answer to the first question is: *very very* diluted. There are actually two levels of dilution. In one level, the *centesimal scale* of dilution, one part of the sub-stance is diluted with a hundred parts of distilled water or ethyl alcohol. This solution is shaken. The poten-tized solution is then further diluted by taking one part and adding it to a hundred parts of water or alcohol. This, too, is shaken, and diluted in a 1:100 ratio, and so on. This process of dilution and succussion is re-peated a number of times to achieve a particular po-tency—each time increases the dilution by a factor of one hundred. The centesimal scale is the most common in the United States, and is represented by the letter *c* after the number of dilutions: 1c for the first dilution (1:100), 2c for the second dilution (1:10,000), and so on. The most common centesimal dilutions are 3c, 6c, 9c, 12c, 30c, 200c, 1,000c, 10,000c, 50,000c, or 100,000c.

The other common level of dilutions is the *decimal scale*. In this instance, the substance is sequentially di-luted in a one-part-to-ten-part ratio. The letter *x* is used to identify decimal potencies: 1x (1:10); 2x (1:100); and so on.

The resulting potentized remedies are then prepared for use in a number of ways, often by adding them to

tiny sugar tablets. Higher potencies are generally reserved for professional use in chronic diseases, and for
treating mental and emotional symptoms. Experience
has shown they act deeper and longer and that fewer
doses are needed. The lower potencies are usually used
for acute or minor conditions and are available over the
counter for self-care.

Classical (Traditional) Homeopathy

Classical homeopathy adheres strictly to the principles
and rules set forth by Hahnemann and his followers.
This tradition dictates that you should use a single
remedy, in the minimum dose, to treat a person and
that a disease and its cure progress in a predictable
manner.

The Single Remedy. In classical homeopathy, you prescribe one remedy at a time because that one remedy is
the most similar to the total symptom picture. This
remedy is called the *simillimum.* By way of contrast,
allopathic medicine often prescribes a number of drugs
at once, each for a different symptom. For example,
you may take a decongestant, cough medicine, and pain
reliever for a simple cold or flu; or a muscle relaxer and
an antiinflammatory for a sports injury; and an antacid,
acid blocker, and tranquilizer for a stress-induced stomach ulcer. Multiple drugs raise the risk of multiple side
effects and drug interactions: they may exaggerate each
other's effects or in some cases even cancel each other
out, either of which outcome can be dangerous. Very
few studies exist to document the safety of multiple-
drug regimens.

The Minimum Dose. Another important principle in homeopathy is that the proper dose of a remedy is the minimum amount required to stimulate a cure. This is the least amount to which your vital force will respond sufficiently. The minimum dose refers, firstly, to the potency of a remedy—you use the lowest potency that will be effective. In the minor or acute illnesses you'll be treating with self-care, low potencies usually suffice (3, 6, or 12x or c); medium potencies are 30 and 200x or c. Anything above 200x or 200c is considered to be high potency and is usually reserved for professional homeopathic treatment of chronic disease or a severe acute disease such as pneumonia, phlebitis (vein inflammation), or a stomach ulcer.

The Single Dose. Related to the minimum dose is the concept of the single dose. In classical homeopathy, once you have chosen the simillimum and its potency, you administer it in a "single dose." This may be one potency in divided doses and given at short intervals; or it may be different potencies given within a few hours of each other. Once this single dose or short course is completed, the treatment is suspended and you wait and watch for a reaction. In some cases of high-potency remedies for chronic disease, a single dose is all that is ever needed, or it may need to be repeated in a few months or years.

The Healing Process: Hering's Law of Cure

When you have prescribed the correct remedy, symptoms disappear (and may reappear) in a predictable order. This order confirms that the correct remedy has been used, and helps you (or your homeopath) determine that a case is progressing well; it also helps predict what will happen next so both you and your homeopath know what to expect. According to this principle, known as Hering's Law of Cure, symptoms disappear:

1) from the inside toward the outside;
2) from the most important organs toward the least important organs, or from the top of the body to the bottom;
3) in the reverse of the chronological order in which they appeared.

Therefore, as part of this healing pattern, a serious internal physical symptom could be transformed into a new minor external symptom, such as a stomach problem giving way to a skin rash; eventually the skin rash disappears as well. Or, in keeping with the top-to-bottom rule, the pattern could express itself by muscle aches moving from the neck down to the legs before disappearing completely.

Since homeopathy believes that chronic disease can be the result of minor surface symptoms such as skin eruptions being driven deeper through drug suppression (such as cortisone creams), older symptoms often reappear as part of the healing process. (This sequence is not to be confused with symptoms disappearing in the reverse order of appearance, in which the symptoms are still present.) Even if new symptoms appear, or old ones reappear, the person generally feels better in spite of them because a cure is in progress, and symptoms are moving in the right direction.

Studies Prove Homeopathic Remedies Work

Homeopaths point to the nearly two hundred years of clinical experience of convinced doctors and satisfied patients. As a group, homeopathic physicians have found they get good results when treating a wide variety of illnesses, especially infectious diseases such as flu and colds, and chronic conditions such as allergies, asthma, migraines, and PMS—conditions with which conventional medicine hasn't had much success. But conventional science does not accept such purely "anecdotal" evidence as proof. Such successes could be due to the placebo effect, or to bias on the part of the practitioners, who naturally tend to evaluate their results favorably. Or, critics say, perhaps patients who have invested their money, time, and trust simply believe and want so badly to get better that they report improvement whether they feel better or not.

Experimental scientific studies do exist, which help correct this lack of proof. The most recent studies aim to be randomized, double-blind, and placebo controlled. This is the "gold standard" of studies, which is considered to be highly rigorous and accurate. The subjects are randomly divided into two groups, one of which gets the active treatment, and the other "control" group gets a placebo. Both subjects and researchers are "blinded": neither knows which group gets which until the study is over. The results of the two groups are then compared to see if there is any difference and, if so, how much. In 1994, the first study that involved homeopathy was published in a peer-reviewed American scientific journal. Jennifer Jacobs, M.D., led the study, which was conducted in Nicaragua and included eighty-one children with acute diarrhea. All the

children received standard antidehydration treatment
for diarrhea, consisting of water containing salt and
sugar. In addition, half the children received homeopathic treatment and half received a placebo. The study
confirmed homeopathy's effectiveness: the recovery
time for children receiving homeopathic treatment was
20 percent faster than those receiving the placebo, reducing the bout of diarrhea by one day. These results
are heartening because diarrhea is the leading cause of
death in developing countries such as Nicaragua. The
study, which appeared in the May issue of *Pediatrics,*
was a milestone for homeopathy in the United States.
According to the *Boston Globe* article on the study,
several specialists said it might prompt physicians to
take another look at homeopathy as a "valid approach
worthy of consideration."

Many studies on homeopathy have been published in
equally prestigious journals in England, France, and
Germany. In 1991, the *British Medical Journal* published an analysis of 107 clinical studies published between 1966 and 1990. The authors found that in 81 of
the experiments, the homeopathic treatments were successful. Even when they included only the 23 studies
that they considered to be of the highest quality, the
vast majority of these (15) showed positive results.

The authors of the analysis, who were nonhomeopathic Dutch physicians, were perplexed by the positive results. But, they said, "based on this evidence, we
would be ready to accept that homeopathy can be effi-
cacious if only the mechanism of action were more
plausible." They also felt that their analysis made a
case for further evaluation "by means of well-per-
formed controlled trials." Of the studies they analyzed

42 were in English-speaking journals; the remainder were mostly German and French journals.

Here's how the results broke down: 13 out of the 19 trials of respiratory infection treatment were effective, 6 out of 7 were positive for other infections, 5 out of 7 were positive for digestive system treatment, 5 out of 5 were successful for hay fever, 5 out of 7 showed accelerated recovery after surgery, 4 out of 6 helped in rheumatological disease, 18 of 20 were beneficial for pain or traumatic injury; and 8 out of 10 worked for mental or psychological problems.

One study by Dr. David Taylor Reilly, a prominent Scottish physician, stands out in particular. It was published in 1986 in a highly respected British medical journal, *The Lancet*. In this double-blind controlled study, Dr. Reilly and his colleagues compared the effects of a homeopathic hay-fever remedy with a placebo. They found that those who received the homeopathic remedy had six times fewer symptoms and were able to cut their use of antihistamines in half.

Another study published in 1989 in the *British Medical Journal* dealt with a rheumatoid disease called "fibromyalgia." This musculoskeletal disease affects an estimated three to six million U.S. citizens. The double-blind, controlled trial was also "crossed over," meaning the treatment lots were switched after one month so the subjects could be compared, not only with each other, but also with themselves. The results were evaluated by a rheumatology professional who was not a homeopath. The study found that the homeopathic remedy provided highly statistically significant improvement in both subjective and objective symptoms.

This study was milestone for homeopathy, because it was published in the official journal of the British Medical Association, which had previously condemned homeopathy along with other nonmainstream medicines. In addition, the patients were first seen by a homeopathic doctor to ensure that they all fit the pattern of symptoms for Rhus toxicodendron, the only homeopathic remedy being tested. This was an important precaution, because homeopathic remedies are selected according to how closely the individual's totality of symptoms matches that of the remedy. When this is not taken into consideration, and studies accept patients who may not fit the symptom pattern, the odds are weighted against showing a beneficial effect.

The problem of individualizing the therapy may have affected the results of a similar earlier British study (in 1986) of fibromyalgia using three homeopathic remedies. According to the published results of this study, there was no significant difference between the effects of homeopathy and placebo. However, when the results were analyzed further, another picture emerged. The subjects whose total symptom patterns matched the homeopathic remedy they received did appear to benefit. This suggests that the subjects who enjoyed no benefits may not have received the correct remedy for their particular case.

A still earlier study, in 1980, again conducted in Britain, showed very positive results for rheumatoid arthritis. In this double-blind controlled study, 82 percent of those receiving the homeopathic remedy enjoyed improvements in their condition versus 21 percent of the control group on placebo. The subjects in this study received remedies that were individually prescribed.

An experiment with osteoarthritis did not fare so well, however, and again homeopaths feel this could have been due in part to incorrect prescribing. Patients

were given Rhus tox or a conventional antiinflammatory painkiller. The painkiller was found to be the
most effective, but the remedy was not individualized,
and Rhus tox is rarely given for osteoarthritis, but
often for rheumatoid arthritis, a very different condition. In addition, a fast-acting conventional drug that
suppresses symptoms was pitted against a homeopathic
remedy that acts slowly to cure a condition—an unfair
comparison.

Other significant positive studies show homeopathy
helps in pain following tooth extraction (76 percent
versus 40 percent for a placebo); reduces vertigo and
nausea; reduces labor time in pregnant women (5.1
hours versus 8.5 hours); and reduces risk of abnormal
labor (11.3 percent versus 40 percent).

There have been two sets of studies conducted on
two over-the-counter homeopathic remedies that also
met with positive results. Two double-blind studies
compared Quietude, a combination of homeopathically
prepared plant extracts that has been popular in France
for twenty years, with diazepam (Valium), the well-
known tranquilizer. The studies were performed on
adults and children who were nervous and suffered
from sleeplessness. They showed that the homeopathic
product increased sleep time, reduced interruptions
during sleep, and reduced nervousness. Both products
relieved insomnia and minor nervous tension 63 percent of the time. However, the homeopathic product
produced no side effects: there was no daytime dizziness, as opposed to 13 percent of the diazepam group;
no daytime drowsiness, but 53 percent of the diazepam
group felt drowsy. In addition, Quietude was better at
reducing children's nightmares, and 74 percent of the
Quietude patients said the product was better than

other treatments, as opposed to 48 percent of the diazepam group who felt this way.

The other group of studies tested Oscillococcinum (ah-sil-oh-kok-SIGH-num), derived from duck heart and liver, for its ability to relieve flu symptoms. All three studies found it to be effective for fever, shivering, and ailing due to flu. One of the studies, conducted in 1985, found that in the group who took the homeopathic product, fever decreased more rapidly—in two days—than in the placebo group; and shivering disappeared by day four. The second controlled study, published in 1989 in the *British Journal of Clinical Pharmacology,* found that 66 percent more of the Oscillococcinum group recovered within forty-eight hours.

Other research supports homeopathy's value in treating infectious diseases. In a French study published in 1987, silica, prepared homeopathically to the 10c potency, stimulated macrophage activity by nearly 70 percent. Macrophages are white cells belonging to the immune defense system that "eat" harmful cells and microorganisms. Homeopathic remedies have also corrected immunological disorders in mice. In other studies, eight out of ten homeopathic remedies tested were able to inhibit the growth of viruses (in chicken embryos) by 50 to 100 percent.

Although we have no large controlled studies as of yet, clinicians working with HIV-infected people have reported that homeopathic remedies help their immune-deficient patients in several ways. They reduce the incidence, length, and severity of opportunistic infections, may slow the progression to ARC or AIDS, help treat acute infections and reduce the need for antibiotics or other drugs, increase the number of T-cells, prevent weight loss, and possibly extend life.

There were encouraging results in a 1992 study conducted on sixty people with retinal problems due to diabetes. In approximately half of the patients taking the homeopathic remedy (Arnica), the eye condition improved; only 1 percent of the subjects receiving placebo improved a like amount. The subjects were evaluated using objective measuring instruments, indicating that homeopathy may prove valuable in helping this group of diabetics preserve their sight.

There is further evidence that homeopathy does not work solely because of the placebo effect. Homeopathic remedies are used successfully on animals and infants, who are less likely to be influenced by placebo. In Germany, poultry farmers are treating their hens with homeopathic remedies instead of antibiotics for coughs, colds, and digestive problems. They thus avoid the harmful drug residues in eggs that are prohibited by German law, and save the $15,000-per-henhouse infection it would cost if they used conventional antibiotics. Farmers also treat their cats, dogs, horses, cattle, and birds homeopathically.

Other animal studies add to the evidence. A 3x potency of Chelidonium lowered cholesterol in rabbits by 25 percent. Microdoses of Arsenicum (10x up to 30x; and 5c up to 15c) helped rats eliminate toxic doses of arsenic from their systems, a study that has important implications for humans who are increasingly exposed to many heavy metals in the environment. And pigs given Caulophyllum had half as many stillbirths as those who received a placebo.

Homeopaths have been reporting good results when

treating infants for common health problems such as teething, colic, eczema, and fever.

Furthermore, the placebo effect does not explain the successes homeopathy enjoyed during the epidemics of cholera, typhoid, yellow fever, and scarlet fever in the 1800s. In addition, homeopathic doses create symptoms in ultrasensitive people during provings—evidence that highly diluted substances do have a biological action. Placebos rarely cause a similar group of symptoms. Finally, homeopathic remedies sometimes cause a temporary exacerbation of symptoms called a "healing crisis." Placebos may relieve symptoms but virtually never worsen them.

How Do Homeopathic Remedies Work?

The potentization procedure produces remedies that are so dilute that according to the known laws of physics and chemistry, they couldn't possibly have any effect. Once you get beyond a certain point—24x or 12c —there is probably not even one single molecule of the original active substance remaining. This point was proven mathematically by an Italian physicist, Amadeo Avogadro, in 1811.

And yet, according to homeopathic doctrine and experience, the more diluted the solution, the more potent it is. This apparent paradox has not yet been satisfactorily explained by scientific standards—a fact that is of secondary importance to homeopaths, who find that the remedies work and see no reason to stop using them simply because we have no proven mechanism as to how they work. Homeopaths point out that pharmacologists would not be able to explain exactly how most conventional drugs work—even aspirin is not fully understood!—but still orthodox medicine believes in them and prescribes them.

However, some plausible explanations do exist, even if they have not been proven and remain largely theoretical. The effects of microdoses have been known for a long time, and there are a number of examples that support the idea that very diluted concentrations of a substance will have a measurable and sometimes profound effect. Science even has a name for this phenomenon: *hormesis*.

As an illustration of hormesis, Michigan State University researchers used microdoses of a fertilizer to stimulate crop production, according to a study published in *Science* magazine. In a dose equivalent to a 9x dilution, the fertilizer increased tomato yield by 30 percent, carrots were 21 percent bigger, and corn yield increased by 25 percent. Another example is the one milligram of acetylcholine diluted in 500,000 gallons of blood that has been shown to lower a cat's blood pressure; an even more dilute solution affects a frog's heart. Our own bodies secrete minute amounts of hormones that have powerful effects. Thyroid hormone is present in our blood at only 1 part per 10 billion—yet this is enough to regulate the rate of our entire metabolism. Many animal studies show that low doses of some substances elicit a beneficial response while high doses are harmful. This phenomenon has been documented to occur with radiation, antibiotics, and heavy metals.

Some homeopaths also point to *pheromones* as an example of individual sensitivity to minute amounts of substances. Pheromones are powerful aromatic hormonelike substances that creatures secrete to attract one another. One molecule of moth pheromone is so potent, it will attract another moth from miles away and trigger a cascade of physical reactions. Though well documented, the exact mechanism for pheromones remains unknown.

However, as Avogadro's work shows, many homeopathic remedies are so diluted, they don't have even one molecule of the substance in them, so hormesis doesn't fully explain their effects. Interestingly, even when the substance is so highly diluted that there are no detectable molecules of it remaining, there are experiments indicating that something is left of the original substance which has an effect visible on a microscopic level.

For example, a renowned French immunologist named Benveniste showed in 1988 and again in 1991 that homeopathically diluted and potentized doses of substances can affect blood cells. His original research in 1988 used an antibody as the homeopathic substance (an antibody is a naturally occurring substance manufactured by the body). The blood cells reacted as if they had been exposed to the full-strength antibody. When published in the scientific journal *Nature*, the study attracted a lot of publicity and became highly controversial. Although his work was replicated by other respected scientists around the world, it was supposedly "debunked" by a fraud expert, a magician (the "Amazing" Randi), and two representatives of the journal who were not immunologists. Homeopaths protested that the debunking itself had serious problems. The debunkers were inexperienced in immunology research and did not test the antibody an adequate number of times (it was effective in one out of four tests); they did not adequately screen blood samples; and they did not allow for the fact that good immunological research is often effective only 30 to 50 percent of the time. Sometime later, Benveniste himself repeated his potentized antibody experiment and 39 percent of the time showed an effect when compared to distilled water. In another set of experiments he used homeopathically diluted *apis* (crushed bees) and found dramatic results.

So, assuming something is going on, how do we explain the effects of a substance that seems, as someone once observed, to be not a drug, but more like the idea of a drug?

The most controversial and intriguing theory, and the one with the most promise, is that these remedies do not work on a physical plane at all and so cannot be measured and analyzed by physical means. Hahnemann believed that dilution and succussion released a spiritlike power that worked on the spiritual level of the vital force in humans. Today we know that formerly invisible, immeasurable, unknowable energy forms do exist, such as electromagnetic radiation and subatomic particles. Magnets exerted their force long before science could explain the mechanism. Physicists are still trying to explain gravity and the nature of matter, still discovering phenomena such as the "strong force" and the "weak force."

Homeopathy, at bottom, is not a physical medicine. It is an energy medicine, as are acupuncture (which has enjoyed increasing acceptance within orthodox medicine for anesthesia, pain relief, and in treating drug withdrawal) and therapeutic touch (which is being taught and offered in major medical institutions because it accelerates healing). Homeopaths believe that although the physical molecules of the original substance may be gone, dilution and succussion leaves something behind—an imprint of its essence, or its energy pattern—that gives it a kind of healing charge. Potentization does not occur if you simply dilute the substance, even if you dilute it repeatedly. Nor does it occur if you only shake the substance vigorously. There is something about each process that builds sequentially upon the other, causing the power to be retained and progressively intensified.

But how does the information in such a minute amount of substance get transferred to the body? Some theorists suggest the repeated succussion creates an electrochemical pattern that is stored in the water carrier and then spreads like liquid crystallization through the body's own water (human bodies are three-fourths water); others say the dilution process triggers an electromagnetic imprinting that directly affects the electromagnetic field of the body.

The new physics, also called "quantum physics" or "quantum mechanics," has made some startling discoveries that may relate to potentization. It tells us that matter (the material world) and energy (the nonmaterial world) are one and the same. Matter is made of molecules and atoms, and atoms are made of subatomic particles. Particles appear to be nothing but nonmaterial waves moving through nonmaterial fields. As one physicist said, "What we used to regard as solid objects are found to be a ghostly mosaic of quivering energy." Once we get down to the level of the subatomic particle, solid matter as we understand it does not exist, and the standard laws of physics do not apply.

Our solid world of trees and streets and books and people only seems solid because we live at a macroscopic level and our senses tell us that all this stuff is solid. But underneath it all, subatomic particles are energetically "dancing" in precise patterns. Thus, it becomes less farfetched to theorize that a homeopathic remedy's "signal" to the vital force may be informational and electromagnetic in nature.

Some research seems to show that if shaken properly, water does retain a "memory" of what was in it. It has a particular molecular order, as does ethyl alcohol to a lesser degree. The molecules tend to group together at room temperature in "flickering clusters." Succussion might affect the vibratory motion in the water or alcohol molecules, raising the vibrational energy by several levels. This could create configurations of molecules specific to a particular medicine. The molecules of the original substance transfer their information to water molecules by transferring a unique energy pattern. It has been proposed that with each dilution and succussion, the information transfer becomes clearer and purer and therefore more effective, like tuning in a radio station more precisely. The "signal" our vital force receives becomes louder and clearer.

Nuclear magnetic resonance technology (NMR), also called "magnetic resonance imaging" (MRI), is able to measure the spin of subatomic particles called "protons." A 1983 study examined twenty-three homeopathic remedies and found that they did possess distinct readings, but a placebo did not. What this early research points to is fairly startling. Homeopathy could be as different from conventional medicine as the new physics is from the old physics. The homeopathic view of disease is more complicated than what is known as "psychosomatic illness." Homeopathy is asking scientists to rewrite chemical and scientific laws and revise the scientific theory on which the entire conventional medical system is based.

It is little wonder that there are still skeptics—especially in the U.S.—due to stubborn resistance, lack of education, vested interest, and failure of motivation. But most blame the absence of a physically provable link between homeopathic remedies and any known disease mechanism. Accepting homeopathy calls for a drastic change in the way one thinks of chemistry. Physicians need to ignore much of what they've learned in medical school about physics and the disease process. They need to broaden the definition of *wellness* to include the physical, mental, and emotional levels. Considering the track record of orthodox medicine, a strong case could be made that medicine has much to learn about health and healing and that the time for such a shift has come.

HOMEOPATHIC MEDICINE	CONVENTIONAL MEDICINE
ILLNESS is an individual expression of imbalance and has important meaning	occurs in well-defined groups based on pathology, and meaning of illness is irrelevant
SYMPTOMS are evidence of disharmony and the person's attempt to restore order	are bad
are analyzed to follow progress of treatment	successful treatment makes them go away
DIAGNOSIS the understanding of the phenomenon of the illness	the search for the structural cause
the whole person is taken into account	
TREATMENT individualized and based on the entire expression of symptoms	based on the pathologic diagnosis
self-care (what the client does) is emphasized	what the doctor does is emphasized
based on *Like cures like* and potentized microdoses of medicines	based on opposing and suppressing symptoms, and high doses of medicine

THREE

. . . .

Homeopathic Self-Care

Most homeopathic care in the U.S. takes place in the home, and most homeopathic remedies are used for self-care. In this chapter you'll learn how to take a case, evaluate it and make a diagnosis, select the appropriate homeopathic remedy, give the remedy, and follow the case. By following these guidelines, you'll be able to effectively and safely treat a variety of minor illnesses and injuries at home, in yourself, your family, and friends.

Taking the Case

Your first step is to assemble the homeopathic symptom picture by "taking the case." This process is a shorter, simpler version of the one used by professional homeopaths. When taking a case, use the chart provided on page 47 to write down your findings (either photocopy it, or copy it by hand).

To take a case, ask yourself or your patient about the following three categories of symptoms and fill in the Case-Taking Chart:

> *General symptoms.* These occur throughout the body and include fatigue, restlessness, relative body heat, pattern of sweat, food desires and aversions; they also include emotional symptoms such as sadness or depression.
> *Particular symptoms.* These are localized to a particular part of the body and include headache, sore throat, skin eruption, or abdominal discomfort.
> *Peculiar symptoms.* These are not usually present in a similar illness, or are just odd. Oftentimes, the peculiar symptoms provide the type of information that allows you to zero in on just the right remedy. Examples would be a burning pain relieved by heat, tooth pain relieved by chewing, or a cough made better by lying down.

Also ask about *modalities*—anything that makes the symptoms better or worse, such as heat, cold, or movement.

Case-Taking Tips

- Let your patient use his or her own words to describe symptoms and use those words in the chart.
- Use open-ended questions to avoid swaying your patient. For example, "When does it feel worse?" is better than "Does the cold make it worse?"

- In some cases you may need to offer suggestions, but make sure you supply several options, such as "Do you feel different during the morning, afternoon, or evening? With cold or heat? With movement or rest?"
- When your patient is a child or, for some other reason, has trouble describing her symptoms in sufficient detail, rely on your observations to supply information. Is she shivering? Feverish? Covered up to her neck with blankets? Tugging at her ears? Do these symptoms seem to get better or worse with changes in the weather, time of day, inside or outside the house?
- Some physical examination will also provide symptom information. For example, taking the temperature, looking into the throat for swelling, redness, or white spots, feeling the temperature of the hands, and so on.
- Realize that you might find it difficult to take your own case. You may feel too ill to be observant or objective. If possible, enlist the aid of someone else to help you assemble your symptom picture.

Before taking a case, you may want to read through some of the descriptions of the conditions and the glossary of the remedies—this will give you a general understanding of the scope and type of information you'll need to compile about symptoms before making a diagnosis and prescribing a remedy. As a further aid, study the sample chart provided on page 48.

CASE-TAKING CHART

Name of Patient: _____

Date: _____

Name of Condition: _____

	Severity	Modalities	Onset
General symptoms (whole body)			
Particular symptoms (local)			
Peculiar symptoms (unusual)			

Remedy & potency prescribed _____

Schedule of Administration _____
Results:

CASE-TAKING CHART

Name of Patient: _____ *Carol* _____

Date: _____ *12/10/95* _____

Name of Condition: _____ *Flu* _____

	Severity	Modalities	Onset

General symptoms   *Lots of aches in muscles.*
   (whole body)   *Feels really weak and tired. Can barely move . . . too weak. Seems very sleepy. No thirst or appetite. Fever is 102°.*

Particular symptoms   *Scratchy throat.*
   (local)   *Mild runny nose (clear). A few coughs, dry, but sleeps OK. Severe headache, worse from moving around (pulsates).*

Peculiar symptoms   *Began slowly over a few days.*
   (unusual)   *Lies there looking dazed & dull. Doesn't even want to watch T.V.*

Remedy & potency prescribed _____ *Gelsemium 30C* _____

Schedule of Administration _____ *3x* _____

Results: *Slowly better. Much more energy by 12/12 & better completely by 12/15.*

   Other school friends had the flu with high fever & were sick for 2 weeks.

Evaluating the Case

You next need to study the case and determine the key symptoms. To help you decide, ask your patient or yourself: which symptoms are the most intense, the most severe, cause the most misery, and limit physical and mental/emotional functioning the most? Also bear in mind that generally, strong or unusual mental/emotional symptoms carry the most weight. For example, your patient may have a cough, a headache, or fever—physical symptoms. But he may also be grieving over the loss of a loved one, or a job, or some other loss that may be connected to the illness. While one person with the flu may enjoy or demand the company of others, another person will be irritable and want to be left alone. One child with an earache will be weepy and cry pitifully, while another child will be angry and hit or throw things. Using a rating system such as a scale of one to three, indicate the severity of each symptom in the appropriate column.

Selecting the Homeopathic Remedy

Now you are ready to begin matching the symptoms of your patient to the symptoms of the remedy. First turn to "The A-to-Z Guide to Common Conditions" and read about the condition that most resembles your patient's. If he or she has an earache, turn to "Earache"; if the symptoms suggest a cold or flu, turn to the section on "Colds" or "Flu." Once you've determined your patient's condition, refer to the homeopathic remedies listed under that condition. In many cases, you will find a remedy that matches simply by referring to these suggestions. If not, write down the ones that provide the closest match and then turn to the "Glossary of Homeopathic Remedies" for additional information about each remedy. Then choose the one that best fits *most* of the symptoms, paying attention to the modalities and personality characteristics as well.

Next, decide on a potency. In homeopathic self-care, the low potencies are generally recommended in either the decimal (x) or centesimal (c) level. These include 6, 12, and 30. The higher the number, the higher the potency, and the quicker and deeper the effect.

Forms of Homeopathic Remedies

Homeopathic remedies are available in several forms, which generally come in a variety of potencies.

Tinctures are alcohol extracts of an original plant substance and are usually applied externally; they are also used as the basis for preparing the various potencies in other forms.

Liquid dilutions generally come in brown glass bottles of 30 milliliters or 60 milliliters. These are usually taken in drops, which are either mixed with water and kept in the mouth for a minute before swallowing, or are placed directly under the tongue.

Triturations are tablets or medicated powders consisting of a sucrose or lactose (milk sugar) base. These are usually used for insolvent substances such as metals. Sold in various sizes (one, two, or four ounces), the remedy is put under the tongue and allowed to dissolve gradually before swallowing, or added to distilled water first.

Granules and globules (pellets) are small spheres made of lactose and sugar that have been impregnated with a potentized dilution of the remedy. Granules are much smaller than globules and resemble cake sprinkles; they are usually used for potencies of 30c and higher.

Taking the Remedy

Because of their unique nature and process of preparation, homeopathic remedies cannot be handled like allopathic medicines. Once out of their container, they can become depotentized and contaminated. To prevent this, avoid touching a remedy with your hands or fingers. Tip the required number of pellets out of the bottle onto a clean piece of plain white paper, or into the bottle cap and then into your mouth.

The preferred method is to place the remedy under your tongue and allow pellets to dissolve slowly, for one to two minutes. This sublingual delivery allows the remedy to be directly absorbed into the bloodstream through the tiny capillaries that line the underside of the tongue. If the remedy is swallowed immediately the whole dose becomes mixed with stomach acid but usually works just as well. A liquid remedy is held in the mouth—as much of it under the tongue as possible—for a minute or two before swallowing.

Do not eat or drink anything for thirty minutes before and after taking the remedy; you may drink bottled or filtered water (chlorine free) during this time. The goal is to have only your natural odors in your mouth when you take the remedy. Although philosophies differ, many homeopaths advise that you avoid coming into contact with camphor or coffee during the course of treatment, and for at least forty-eight hours after the last dose. These substances may antidote the remedy, negating its effects and causing your symptoms to return. Camphor is found in many cosmetics and skin creams, lip balms, and cold remedies such as chest rubs. Caffeine is found in coffee and nonherbal teas (even decaffeinated still contains some caffeine), colas, chocolate, and many drugs.

Some homeopaths also advise you to avoid mint, menthol, eucalyptus, and other strong-smelling herbs— even to the point of switching from ordinary toothpaste to baking soda or a special homeopathic toothpaste. These substances do not always necessarily interact with a homeopathic remedy, so if you should for some reason come into contact with one of them, monitor yourself for any changes or return of symptoms. You may be able to repeat the original remedy and again achieve good results, or you may need to change to another remedy. Other homeopaths advise that you do not use toothpaste or mouthwash for at least one hour before and after taking the remedy because of their aromatic ingredients, such as mint.

In addition, you should avoid taking any allopathic drugs (prescription or over-the-counter) during treatment because they may interfere with the effectiveness of the homeopathic remedy. Check with your homeopath, if you are seeing one, to be sure. Also, you should never discontinue any prescribed medication without consulting your treating physician in advance.

Storing and Handling Homeopathic Remedies

You can store your homeopathic remedies indefinitely if they have been prepared and bottled properly. However, you need to follow a few basic rules to maintain their potency and avoid contamination.

- Keep them in an airtight container, away from heat, sunlight, and strong-smelling substances such as perfume, mothballs, or camphor that could contaminate them. They may be kept in a room-temperature cupboard, not refrigerated, because refrigerators tend to hold a variety of strong odors.
- Do not transfer the remedy to another container.
- Keep the bottle tightly capped when not in use and close it immediately after taking the remedy.
- Open one bottle at the time to prevent cross-potentization.
- If, during administration, extra pills fall out of the bottle, do not return them to the container—throw them away.

Buying the Remedy

Homeopathic remedies are becoming increasingly available in drugstores, health food stores, and homeopathic drugstores. If there is no outlet near you, you may buy them by mail; see the "Resources" section of this book for the largest and most reputable suppliers.

Because ordering each remedy by mail (or even going directly to a retail supplier) can result in undesirable delays in treatment, it is recommended that you purchase or assemble your own homeopathic remedy kit in 12 or 30c potency. This way, you have the most commonly called-for remedies always on hand the moment you need them. Kits come in a variety of sizes, to which you can add at any time. If possible, have on hand a *full homeopathic kit,* consisting of all of the remedies in the glossary section of this book. If you'd rather start small, it is recommended that you have a kit that contains at least the following remedies:

Basic Homeopathic Remedy Kit

Aconite
Arnica montana
Arsenicum album
Belladonna
Bryonia alba
Chamomilla
Ferrum phosphoricum
Gelsemium
Hepar sulphuricum
Hypericum perforatum
Ignatia imara
Mercurius vivas
Nux vomica
Pulsatilla
Rhus toxicodendron

Combination Remedies. If, after taking and evaluating a case, you are still unsure of the appropriate single remedy, or if you are not ready to invest in a remedy kit, combination remedies are an excellent way to get your feet wet. These products usually consist of three or more low-potency remedies (3x to 12x is common) combined in a single liquid or tablet. The remedies included are those that are commonly used for a specific condition, and the products are usually named for the specific condition such as flu, insomnia, cough, hay fever, or PMS. Combination remedies are readily available at health food stores and pharmacies and are easy to prescribe, since they don't require much effort or knowledge to select. The results are not as specific, since the remedy is not as specific to the case, but some degree of positive result is almost guaranteed. This way, you can gradually build your confidence in homeopathy and your ability to use it in acute self-care situations.

Dosage Frequency: Follow the Rule of Three

Since the frequency of dosage of a homeopathic remedy depends on the severity of the symptoms, you should not necessarily follow the directions on the remedy's container. Because the FDA has refused to fully understand homeopathic remedies, its regulations have imposed a standard set of printed instructions, and these do not reflect their usage in the practical world. Paying close attention to changes in symptoms is your only true guide as to how frequently a homeopathic remedy should be given.

General stepwise guidelines for dosage follow the "Rule of Three," which is a simple, easy way to determine how much of a remedy is appropriate under varying circumstances. There are three levels of severity and three corresponding intensities of dosage. Depending on the form the remedy comes in, each dose consists of:

Drops: 5–10
Tablets: 2–3
Globules: 2–3
Granules: 15–20

The Rule of Three is summarized in chart form below. The more severe the symptoms, the more frequently you should give the remedy. In each case, you should stop medication after up to three doses have been given for that day, and wait. If there is improvement, continue with that remedy, but give it less frequently, as indicated in the chart. If there is *marked* improvement, stop the remedy entirely. This means the body's healing process has been triggered sufficiently, and giving more remedy is not only unnecessary, it could stop the recovery process or exaggerate the symptoms.

The Rule of Three—Dosage Guidelines

SEVERE SYMPTOMS

Every one half to one hour for 3 doses, and then . . .	Repeat as necessary for up to one day until symptoms improve to mild or moderate

MODERATE SYMPTOMS

One dose every 3 hours for one day, and then . . .	Repeat as necessary for up to one day until symptoms improve to mild

MILD SYMPTOMS

One dose every 6 hours	Repeat as necessary up to 10 days until symptoms disappear

If there is no improvement whatsoever after the first six doses, you have probably chosen the wrong remedy. You should reevaluate the case, checking the information under both the Condition and Remedy listings. If you feel your choice is still correct, try another three to six doses of the same remedy. If you have doubts, move down the list of recommended remedies and choose the next one that best fits the case and repeat the dosing process. If the second remedy is not working, you may want to try a third. Or, if the case is not urgent, you also may decide to stop medication and let nature take its course.

If it is an urgent case, however, or if the person is getting worse, stop the remedy and seek professional help. The homeopathic remedy will not be harmful, but if it doesn't help, why continue to give it? Continuing the wrong medication may only complicate the symptom picture, making it more difficult to evaluate and treat.

As you treat yourself or another person, be sure to write down each step you've taken and why you've taken it, as well as the results. Also make a note of any improvement that occurs if you do not prescribe anything, but follow only the suggestions for General Homeopathic Home Care. Keep your notes along with the symptom chart as part of the family's home health file. An ongoing health file provides you with a valuable record and better enables you to accurately prescribe the correct remedy. If a certain type of illness recurs after a few years, you can check through the file to see if the symptom pattern is the same and what remedy was used. The successful treatment of acute illness in the home may take on a pattern and you will learn the acute remedies for each family member's coughs, fe-

vers, diarrhea, hay fever, and so on. This information
will also be invaluable to a professional homeopath, if
you decide to have a chronic illness treated homeopathically.

In many instances, one or just a few dosages may be
all that's needed to trigger the healing process. If there
is a relapse soon after the initial improvement, you may
repeat the same remedy, but first make sure the symptom picture really is the same as during the original
illness.

Sometimes the correct remedy causes a slight aggravation of symptoms. This usually is limited to chronic
illness being treated with a high-potency (200c and up)
constitutional remedy. But it may also occur during an
acute illness, and you should be prepared for it. This
"healing crisis" may show itself, for example, as a profuse nasal discharge in a cold, or diarrhea in the flu;
emotional symptoms such as weeping are also not unheard of. These should be temporary and last no more
than twenty-four to forty-eight hours, if the remedy
was correctly selected.

Also bear in mind Hering's Law of Cure (see Chapter
2) when evaluating the effectiveness of a remedy. A
change in symptoms doesn't necessarily call for a
change in remedies. For example, you may have taken a
remedy for a chest cold with a cough. If your chest
symptoms improve, but now you sneeze and have a
runny nose—that's a sign that healing has begun. The
symptoms have moved upward in the body and have
gone from affecting a deep organ to a more superficial
one.

Study Groups

If you wish to deepen your understanding and sharpen your skills, there are many books and cassette tapes, and several videotapes and study courses on homeopathy available (see "Resources" section).

Another possibility is to join or start a homeopathic study group. The National Center for Homeopathy will send you a list of existing groups upon request. Such informal study groups are part of the long tradition of homeopathy, even among faculty and students of homeopathic schools. Participating in such a group allows you to share thoughts, experiences, and questions relating to homeopathy. Members teach each other and keep each other informed about the best new books, magazine articles, and homeopathic journals. They also provide psychological support for like-minded individuals who swim against the current tide of conventional medical care. Lay groups may invite homeopaths to lecture, and also invite the general public to attend and so spread the word about this little-understood form of remedy.

FOUR

. . . .

Seeing a Professional Homeopath

Although this is primarily a book that teaches you how to use homeopathic remedies to treat minor everyday conditions, you may also want to know what a skilled homeopath can do, how to find one, and what to expect under a homeopath's care.

In general, professional care is appropriate and preferable if self-care hasn't worked sufficiently or if you want to go deeper and treat a serious chronic condition. You may also feel safer and more confident practicing self-care if you have an established relationship with a homeopath whom you trust. That way, you have someone who knows you (or whomever you are treating) and with whom you can check to see if you are doing the right thing.

Finding a Homeopathic Practitioner

Unfortunately, there are still relatively few practicing homeopaths in the U.S. It is estimated that half of the homeopaths in this country are licensed medical doctors, many of whom have grown disillusioned with allopathic medicine and have "converted" to homeopathy.

Dana Ullman, president of the Foundation for Homeopathic Education and Research, did a research survey in 1990 and estimated that there were one to two thousand medical doctors and osteopaths practicing homeopathy. In addition, there were one to two thousand other licensed professionals (naturopathic physicians, dentists, podiatrists, veterinarians, physician assistants, nurse practitioners, nurse midwives, nurses, chiropractors, and acupuncturists) who were using homeopathic remedies in their practice. Ullman also estimated there were probably less than a hundred active lay practitioners. However, the legal status of lay practitioners is uncertain, since homeopathic drugs are considered to be over-the-counter medications and so prescribing them is officially regarded as the practice of medicine.

The more serious or disabling the illness, the greater the need for a highly trained and skilled practitioner. A *medical doctor (M.D.)* who practices homeopathy has gone through years of rigorous education and training and has the background to recognize severe pathology (disease) and choose the best course of therapy. A *doctor of osteopathy (D.O.)* has had medical training similar to that of an M.D., but focusing more on the functioning of the musculoskeletal system, and how it interacts with the rest of the body. As is the case with M.D.'s, osteopaths are fully licensed to practice medicine in all fifty states. Increasingly over the years, D.O. training and practice has come to be the same as that of M.D.'s.

A *naturopathic doctor (N.D.)* has completed four years of graduate training, available at two accredited U.S. colleges. Naturopathic training includes extensive understanding of physiology and pathology, but is based on natural medicines such as nutrition, herbs, stress management, and massage or physical manipulation. N.D.'s have the best formal homeopathic education in the U.S. and are supervised in their training clinics, but have no hospital training. Naturopaths have a qualifying exam in homeopathy that confers a diplomate status of the Homeopathic Academy of Naturopathic Physicians (DHANP). As of this writing, naturopaths are licensed in a number of states: Washington, Utah, Oregon, Montana, Hawaii, Florida, Connecticut, Arizona, and Alaska. Idaho, District of Columbia, and North Carolina have "right to practice" laws for naturopaths. In several other states legislation is pending to license naturopaths.

The best way to find a reputable homeopath is through word of mouth from friends or relatives, through a reputable health practitioner, or by contacting any of the homeopathic organizations (listed in the "Resources" section of this book) for a referral.

Depending on where you live, you may not have a tremendous amount of choice in homeopathic practitioners. However, be sure to ask about their credentials. Find out:

- Where the homeopath studied homeopathy and for how long: There are currently no accredited medical schools in the U.S. devoted exclusively to homeopathy. Since homeopathic education takes place outside the conventional medical-school system, homeopaths are likely to have irregular patterns of education. Generally, the more study time the better, and a homeopath should usually have a total of at least five hundred hours of training. This may occur either through seminars, on-site and home-study training programs, or as part of the curriculum of a naturopathic college. The most sophisticated and comprehensive programs are given by the International Foundation for Homeopathy and the Hahnemann College (see "Resources" section of this book). A homeopath should also continue his or her education after a formal training program has been completed, through seminars, workshops, home-study groups, and so on.

- How long the homeopath has been in practice: Ask specifically how much of his or her time has been devoted exclusively to homeopathy. Obviously, the more experienced homeopath is usually more skilled. It takes many years to become familiar with the symptom patterns of the various medicines, and to develop the art of prescribing. A seasoned, experienced homeopath with a relatively small amount of formal training will be a more able practitioner than a freshly minted homeopath just out of a two-thousand-hour comprehensive program in homeopathy.

- If he or she belongs to any professional homeopathic associations: Are they a member of the American Institute of Homeopathy (AIH)? If they are a diplomate of this organization, it means they have taken a nationally recognized qualifying exam and thus meet certain standards. Being a diplomate of homeopathy (Dt.H.) is a plus, but not being one is not a minus. If you are seeing a naturopath find out if he or she is a member of the American Association of Naturopathic Physicians.

• Are they licensed to practice in your state? Medical doctors can practice homeopathy in any state, but only three states (Arizona, Connecticut, and Nevada) issue licenses specifically for homeopathic practice. If you go to another type of health professional for homeopathy, make sure they are licensed in their profession.

The First Visit: Taking the Case

A visit to a homeopathic physician is quite different from a visit to any other type of doctor, especially an allopathic one. You will get a physical examination consisting of anything from a routine general exam to a directed physical exam of the most important problems. If you have recently had multiple exams and tests, your homeopath may just collect those records and focus on the interview part. Some homeopaths feel if a trusted colleague has just examined the person and found no obvious physical changes, it is not necessary to repeat the exam.

Some homeopaths will also order laboratory tests, such as blood tests, urinalysis, X-rays, and referral visits to trusted specialists to clarify various diagnostic issues.

But the real departure comes with the *case taking*—a process that is similar to the one described in Chapter 3, "Homeopathic Self-Care," but much more detailed.

Your interview may last from one to two hours, and in some complicated cases may last even longer. Your homeopath will not only ask about your major symptom, or complaint, but also about minor accompanying symptoms and past symptoms. Be prepared to talk about the character of your symptoms—these include the physical, mental, and emotional planes. Since illness is often a landmark for important life events, your homeopath will likely investigate the time around the onset of the illness as a possible window to cause and cure.

In addition, your homeopath will find out about you as a person: how you generally like to spend your time, how much sleep you get, whether you are an early or late riser, how you get along with other people, if you spend much time alone, what kind of weather you like, and where you have lived in the past and why. Your family health history is very important and is usually taken in great detail. Finally, your own past medical history is of great importance and often reveals the general pattern of illness in your life along with signposts that reveal a great deal.

Once he or she has taken your case, your homeopath will discuss with you your desired goals for homeopathic treatment and what to expect. You will discuss how deeply it is possible for the treatment to go, what is the likely outcome of the treatment, how long the treatment and cure will take, how long the beneficial effects will last.

Some symptoms may be treated directly by removing an external cause—living habits, environmental exposure, stress and worry. This might be all the "treatment" you need, and your homeopath will help you discover and correct the factors, if possible. If they can-

not be removed or only incompletely removed, you
may together decide to look for a mild remedy that will
strengthen you and help you better withstand the situation, and prevent a serious chronic disease from developing.

In some cases, your homeopath will also discuss with
you the possibility that your condition may be too serious or advanced to be treated by homeopathy alone.
You may be referred to another practitioner for treatment; you may then add homeopathic remedies to restore balance, treat the underlying disease, prevent a
recurrence, and speed recovery from allopathic treatment. However, most cases fall somewhere in between
these two extremes, and will respond favorably to the
right homeopathic remedy.

The Homeopathic Diagnosis: Choosing the Right Remedy

Using the detailed results of the case-taking as raw material, your homeopath next forms an analytic picture
of your condition. This process usually begins during
the visit itself. Often while writing everything down
about your case, the homeopath begins looking up your
symptoms in the various homeopathic reference books
he or she keeps in the office. (Some homeopaths incorporate the use of computer programs to narrow down
the remedy choices.) In complicated cases more study
may be required, so the homeopath will advise you
about the remedy in a few days.

Diagnosis and Evaluation. Then your homeopath will
evaluate the relative intensity of your symptoms based

on a number of factors, including how much they are bothering you or interfering with your life and your ability to function. He or she will consider the depth of your symptoms. As explained in Chapter 3, there is an established hierarchy of importance in homeopathy: general and mental problems carry the most weight; then emotional symptoms; and finally physical symptoms, with vital organs being more significant than superficial organs. Out of this process will grow a list of "key symptoms"—the four or five that stand out the most sharply and that will guide the process of selecting the single remedy that most closely matches your totality of symptoms.

Remedy Selection. An experienced, knowledgeable homeopath will by this point in the analysis have a sense of the essence of your disease. He or she will also be familiar with the basic patterns of hundreds of homeopathic drugs, and thus have a sense of the right remedy, or have several strong possibilities in mind. But it is impossible to memorize *all* the symptoms contained in the remedy's symptom picture obtained from the provings. So the homeopath uses the Repertory as a guide in matching the remedy to the symptoms. The Repertory is an alphabetical cross-index of symptoms; the homeopath looks up the symptom and goes through the accompanying list of remedies that cause and cure that symptom. Once the repertorization is complete, the homeopath will usually narrow the choice of remedies to just a few. Further questioning of the patient and additional study in the *Materia Medica* solidifies the choice of the simillimum.

Although the process of selecting the right remedy is methodical and systematic, a sensitive homeopath will

also allow intuition and inspirational insight to guide
him or her in making the final choice. Your personality
also becomes a factor when choosing among two or
possibly three remedies that seem to be a good match.
Personality is one of the most individualizing and distinguishing characteristics of each person, and so it becomes a "divining rod" leading to effective remedy
selection. For example, a person's total symptom picture might indicate either Lachesis or Pulsatilla. If the
person is slow and gentle rather than quick and boister-
ous, then the best choice would be Pulsatilla, because
this remedy is rarely appropriate for a loud, energetic
person. However, it is always the symptoms that arise
during times of distress—and not normal behaviors—
that are crucial in remedy selection.

The process of selecting a single remedy, which is the
goal of the classical homeopath, is the most difficult
aspect of homeopathy. Your homeopath may need to
ask you more questions to get more information, often
about symptoms or modalities that are peculiar or idio-
syncratic, to finally end up with a match that comes
satisfactorily close. Nonclassical homeopaths, on the
other hand, will prescribe several remedies in an attempt to cover all your symptoms.

Choosing the Right Potency

Most homeopaths use a wide range of potencies and
prescribe them according to each individual case. Doses
start at what are called "crude" doses or tinctures, up
to potencies as high as the hundred thousandth.

When homeopathy first became popular in the first

half of the nineteenth century, homeopaths often used tinctures or low (weak) potencies. Hahnemann himself rarely used anything higher (stronger) than the two hundredth, and some sources believe he limited himself to the thirtieth. Today, some homeopaths still limit their prescribing to the lower potencies (between 6 and 30). This is still homeopathy, although other homeopaths report spectacular results with high potencies. The key to prescribing is the Law of Similars, not the level of potency.

(Remember, the more potent the remedy, the less of the original substance it contains.)

Some homeopaths theorize that higher potencies are needed today because times have changed and so has the nature of our illnesses. It may be that the suppressive allopathic drugs we have been taking have driven our illnesses deeper, or our polluted environment effects our health and our ability to respond to the lower potencies.

Homeopaths who use high potencies tend to use them for illnesses that are predominantly mental or emotional in nature, because they can better reach the immaterial plane of the disease. Physical or organic illness—symptoms that exist on a more material plane—respond to low or medium potencies. When there is severe organic illness, or when treating older people, most homeopaths are careful to restrict potencies to the two hundredth or lower, to avoid stimulating the vital force more than the patient can deal with. Children do well with higher potencies, unless there is deep chronic disease, in which case the two-hundredth potency rule again applies.

Taking the Remedy

Your homeopath may administer the remedy in the office and/or give you some to take home with you. Your homeopath may supply you with the remedy from his or her stock, or write you a prescription to be filled by a pharmacy, or recommend an over-the-counter homeopathic remedy sold in pharmacies or health food stores. You may order hard-to-find remedies from a number of large homeopathic pharmaceutical companies with toll-free 800 numbers, or from small specialized pharmacies.

The dosing schedule will depend upon the nature of your symptoms, the goal of the therapy, and how you respond to the remedy. See Chapter 3, "Homeopathic Self-Care," for information about how to take, handle, and store homeopathic remedies.

What to Expect During Treatment

Your homeopath's goal is to promote gentle healing of your disease or condition. There are several common possible outcomes of homeopathic treatment, which your homeopath will evaluate during the course of your treatment and recovery.

1. It's not unusual to experience a noticeable improvement soon after the first dose. A clear improvement in the symptoms of an acute illness can be expected within thirty minutes to three or four hours. Sometimes a sense of well-being or general relief appears almost instanta-

neously. As time goes on, you experience a steady improvement.

2. You may at first experience a temporary aggravation of your existing symptoms after taking a remedy. A slight aggravation is to be considered a positive sign that a cure is under way, and that you will soon feel better.

3. Another positive scenario is for you to undergo a "healing crisis," during which new symptoms appear on the way to your cure. This is common in people being treated with a very potent constitutional remedy for a deep-seated and long-standing chronic condition. Old, long-buried symptoms may reappear, such as skin conditions (rashes, acne), aches and pains, or mental changes. These are temporary and you should avoid the temptation to treat these symptoms allopathically, since the suppression of these symptoms is probably what led to the more serious chronic condition you have now. As long as they appear following Hering's Law of Cure—that is, in reverse of the order of their original appearance—they are a positive, if uncomfortable, sign of progress toward a permanent cure. (See Chapter 2.)

4. You may experience no change, or a worsening of your signs and symptoms. This indicates that the remedy was not the simillimum. Your homeopath needs to reevaluate your case and prescribe a different remedy. Your homeopath may decide that a deep-acting constitutional remedy needs to be given first to assist you in reaching a level where the acute remedy is effective.

5. Another possible reaction is for new symptoms

to appear. This may be a part of the "healing crisis" described above; or it may be a "proving symptom" on the way toward a cure; or it may represent a deepening of the illness (sinus trouble deepening to bronchitis with symptoms of cough and fever). The new symptoms will gradually disappear and are best left untreated. But if they are distressing, your homeopath may administer an antidote. You will also require an antidote if, according to Hering's Law, the symptoms go in the wrong direction, for example from external to internal, or bottom to top.

In a simple acute case, generally, the more severe your symptoms, the more often the remedy is repeated, until improvement is such that you reduce the frequency, and then stop when symptoms are gone. Sometimes only a few days' therapy is needed. In other cases, you may need to take a remedy for several weeks. But if there is no underlying chronic disease, a relapse or return of symptoms usually does not occur. Sometimes a remedy need be given only once, or every few months, or again in a few years. How you respond, and what homeopathic remedy can do, in part depends on your constitution and the skills of the homeopath.

Most homeopaths use a two-pronged approach and prescribe soothing remedies that fit the symptoms of an acute crisis, and when your crisis is over, prescribe a constitutional remedy to work on your underlying disease. When another crisis occurs, he or she may decide to treat that, and then return to the deep-acting constitutional therapy again. This zigzag approach of focusing alternately on acute to chronic and back again continues until your crises grow milder and less frequent and your homeopath detects signs that you have thrown off the underlying chronic disease. Other homeopaths prefer to stick to the single constitutional remedy throughout the course of treatment.

If you have a disease that is very advanced, it may be incurable, even in the hands of the best homeopaths. In this instance your homeopath will try to soothe your symptoms by using lower potencies. You may need to repeat the remedy regularly for a specific period, until the potency has done as much as it can. Then you may move to a higher potency to continue the treatment. Your homeopath may increase the potency in a gradual stepwise fashion through the entire range of potencies for a particular remedy. If your symptom picture changes, your homeopath will take your case again and prescribe a new simillimum.

Follow-up

Acute illnesses generally require minimal follow-up because, depending on their severity, your symptoms will go away within three to forty-eight hours. In chronic disease, however, routine follow-up visits and phone calls are required to monitor and evaluate your case. After your initial visit, you usually need to see your homeopath again every four to six weeks. This may change after two to three visits, according to your progress.

During this follow-up period, you will need to take responsibility for monitoring and perhaps cataloging your symptoms. Your homeopath will instruct you about noting and reporting any dramatic changes, such as the improvement or aggravation of symptoms, or the appearance of new and distressing symptoms. Such events usually indicate you should stop the remedy and call the homeopath for advice, because it is assumed they are reactions to the remedy until this possibility has been ruled out.

Above all, do not medicate yourself or go to an allopathic doctor for treatment of a new symptom without consulting with your homeopathic practitioner first; you should give homeopathy a chance to resolve it. For example, if you are being treated homeopathically for migraine headache and develop a rash, do not go to a dermatologist without first having your homeopath evaluate the symptom.

Cost

Since homeopathy is the practice of medicine, your costs are reimbursed to whatever extent your health plan covers the type of licensed practitioner you are seeing. Many homeopaths participate in "preferred provider" plans, including Blue Cross and Blue Shield; there are few, if any, who are part of HMOs. Homeopaths usually do not accept Medicaid payment because the reimbursement is too small. You should be aware that homeopathic physicians are by and large underpaid for the time they devote to patients: insurance companies assume that an initial visit takes less time than the one to two hours that homeopaths spend; follow-up visits are also underestimated and therefore underpaid.

Homeopaths generally charge fees comparable to those of their nonhomeopathic counterparts, but homeopathic care is ultimately more cost effective. For one thing, there is less need for expensive, invasive diagnosis and treatment. Although homeopaths will often order tests when needed to identify serious physical changes in the body, the need for such tests is decreased over time. Homeopaths do not need to go to the extreme lengths that allopaths go to chase down unlikely causes of symptoms, because natural medicine encourages normal function and cannot cover up important disease that needs diagnosis.

In addition, the need for treatment diminishes over time because homeopathy seeks to heal rather than encourage dependency on tests and drugs that cause side effects, weaken the system, worsen the disease, and lead to more and more doctor visits.

Homeopathy as Complementary Health Care

Some homeopaths feel that all you really need to properly treat an illness is the right homeopathic remedy. But this position is felt by most to be too extreme, and almost allopathic in its faith in medicine as the be-all and end-all. Many homeopaths, rather, talk to patients about their health habits as part of their overall health plan; a good number also feel that, depending on a variety of factors, other natural healing modalities help when appropriately applied; and most will also agree that in certain instances allopathic treatment also has its place.

Healthy Habits are important because the first rule in homeopathy is to "remove all obstacles to a cure." That's why most practitioners will act as health counselors and talk about the importance of nourishment on all three planes of existence. Homeopaths will often advise about physical nourishment, which includes diet, exercise, rest, and vacation time; emotional nourishment, which includes relationships with other people and the free flow of feelings as the juice of life; and mental or spiritual nourishment, which includes learning, community involvement, and our relationship to the infinite of life and death.

For example, many homeopaths themselves eat a vegetarian or macrobiotic diet and encourage their patients to eat a diet rich in vegetables and fruit, whole grains and fiber; and low in fat, sugar, and animal products. Exercise has many physical and psychological health benefits. One of the most important things homeopaths cope with in their patients is overwork—people today are overscheduled and run themselves ragged to make ends meet. Rest and vacations allow us to recuperate from the day's and year's efforts. Part of the tragedy of allopathy is that by suppressing symptoms we can continue to work and thus get sicker by pretending we are well when we are not.

While improving these aspects of our existence can set the stage for health and healing, poor habits may be related to deep issues and be part of the pattern of the total symptom picture. Homeopaths acknowledge that we may not be able to stop eating junk food, or smoking, or drinking, because our disease pattern includes that of various addictive behaviors. We, too, must understand that such changes may not be achievable just by deciding we want to make them, but that homeopathic treatment will help create a landscape in which such changes can more easily be made and be mutually reinforcing.

Other Natural Health Systems include chiropractic, acupuncture and Chinese herbs (traditional Chinese medicine or TCM), herbalism, naturopathy, osteopathy, physical therapy, vitamin and mineral therapy, stress reduction and meditation, and faith healing. These can all be wonderful when appropriately applied, and all can to some degree be successfully used along with homeopathy.

However, it is usually not advisable to mix systems that are complete by themselves and can stand alone, such as TCM. It's best to choose one major system and one primary practitioner to provide, oversee, and coordinate your care. Alternating or simultaneously using more than one vigorous healing system can confuse the bodymind. For clarity of purpose, it is preferable to focus on one form, to become committed to it, and to do it well. This means understanding the basic principles and philosophy, learning about the most common useful remedies, and giving them a chance to work. Then, if you and your practitioner are not satisfied with the results, you should consider trying another modality, either for a particular problem, or for your primary care. For example, you could use homeopathy together with physical therapy to treat a herniated disc in your spine; or homeopathy along with chiropractic to cure a chronic lower back problem. But it is not effective or systematic to impulsively or casually graze in a smorgasbord of health care systems—to pull something off the shelf like a pop-top can or flavor of the month. Such a superficial unfocused approach can only bring superficial results.

Combining with Allopathic Medicine. Homeopaths differ in their attitudes toward allopathic medicine. Many are flexible in their approach and view the two forms as complementary—each is effective when used appropriately. Just as conventional medicine has it limits, so does homeopathy, so why not use the best of both?

Allopathy gets incomparable results, for example, when you have extensive trauma, such as a broken arm that needs to be set and immobilized, or lacerations or wounds, which need to be treated surgically before proper healing can take place. Congenital abnormalities require surgery to put things in place so the person has the physical equipment to function more normally. But homeopathy can relieve the ill effects of surgery, reduce the need for postoperative painkillers, and reduce swelling and speed healing. Homeopathic remedies can also be used preoperatively to prepare you for surgery, and are particularly common in dental surgery, both pre- and postop.

In other cases, homeopathy may be able to delay or avoid surgery, by healing or palliation. For example, women may be cured of uterine fibroid tumors or cysts; or cervical dysplasia (a precancerous condition) may be reversed through homeopathic remedies. Children with chronic ear infections may avoid having drainage tubes surgically implanted, or avoid multiple courses of antibiotics. Men may get enough relief from benign prostate enlargement to avoid surgical removal, a boon in elderly men who are at high risk for surgical complications, including impotence and incontinence. Skin warts, cysts, and painful corns also respond well to homeopathy.

Nontraumatic, nonsurgical emergencies also require allopathic techniques. For example, meningitis, an infection of the brain and spinal cord, can lead to brain damage, disability, and death unless immediate antibiotic treatment is administered. A life-threatening

asthma attack may be best treated with allopathic medication in an emergency room. But again, homeopathic
remedies can be administered on the way to the hospital or after the heroic treatment to accelerate healing
and increase your body's resistance and ability to respond to future crises or infections.

In the case of an advanced chronic disease such as
cancer, diabetes, emphysema, or heart disease, homeopathy may be able to minimize pain, slow the progress
of the disease, and lessen the adverse effects of allopathic treatment. When such diseases progress beyond
a certain stage, it is doubtful that any kind of medical
treatment could effect a cure; however, many appar-
ently terminal patients have lived far longer than pre-
dicted when given homeopathic care. Other incurable
cases include people who have been on strong allopathic drugs for a long time, people with long-term serious mental disorders such as schizophrenia, or those
who have suffered the removal or loss of an important
organ. However, such cases may still be helped, if not
completely cured, by homeopathic treatment.

Homeopaths often see people for whom allopathy
has failed. Sick people turn to alternative methods
when "all else" has failed, and their disease is very advanced. Amazingly, homeopathy often can help in such
cases. But the sequence should be reversed: Homeopaths feel it is best to try homeopathy's gentle approach
first. If homeopathy fails after a reasonable amount of
time, or if the patient is very uncomfortable, debili-
tated, or at risk, then it is reasonable to turn to allopathy, which is much riskier, and harsher, on the person.

Although mainstream medicine is still skeptical of
homeopathy, the American Medical Association no
longer officially condemns it. If you are not ready to

leave the care of your established allopathic physician, or if you have a serious condition that still requires allopathic care, you should talk about your interest in homeopathy with him or her. Whether you use homeopathic self-care or decide to be treated by a licensed professional homeopath, an open discussion with your doctor can benefit you both. Many allopathic physicians were surprised and caught off guard when a 1993 survey showed that one third of Americans used alternative care, indicating a well founded reluctance on the part of patients to share this information with their doctors.

This long overdue wake-up call for the conventional medical establishment means it is less likely you will be rebuffed, or ignored, or patronized, when talking about "alternatives" such as homeopathy. You owe it to your doctor to inform him or her about your other health practices and interests; and he or she owes it to you to listen with an open mind. Show your doctor this book and point out the evidence that homeopathy works. Remember, most of the positive studies appeared in journals published outside the U.S., often in languages other than English, and part of the problem has been that doctors in this country are simply not educated about homeopathy. As informed, active patients, we have the power to help our doctors learn about homeopathic medicine; encourage them to suggest these safe, effective over-the-counter remedies instead of allopathic ones to other patients; and perhaps convince them to convert to homeopathy themselves.

. . . .

PART II

The A-to-Z Guide to Common Conditions and Their Homeopathic Treatment

ABDOMINAL PAIN AND INDIGESTION

Most abdominal pain is due to simple indigestion, whose symptoms include "heartburn," nausea, burping, and intestinal gas, sometimes accompanied by pain. Indigestion may result from eating too much or too fast, an overindulgence in fatty foods, or may be traced to a single food that "doesn't agree with you." Emotional stress may initiate or worsen digestive problems. Abdominal pain and indigestion are also signs of gastroenteritis (inflammation of the stomach or intestinal lining), or of food poisoning, in which a toxic substance such as a pesticide, or spoiled or contaminated food, has inadvertently been consumed. Serious conditions involving abdominal pain include appendicitis, intestinal obstruction, and diseases of the gallbladder, pancreas, and intestines. Vague chronic or recurring abdominal pains in women may be due to pelvic infection or abnormal pregnancy. Chronic abdominal pain, especially if accompanied by other symptoms, should be evaluated by a professional.

See also "Diarrhea, "Vomiting," or "Fever," if they accompany the indigestion.

General Homeopathic Home Care

- Drink plenty of room-temperature beverages.
- Eat small, bland, easily digestible meals such as white rice with overcooked steamed or boiled vegetables; low-fat soup with overcooked vegetables and rice or noodles; thin oatmeal; rice water (make rice as usual but use two to three times the normal amount of water, then drain the water and drink it); skinless boiled or baked potatoes, with low-fat yogurt instead of butter.
- Avoid foods that aggravate symptoms: coffee, alcohol, fatty or fried foods, spices, and raw fruits and vegetables except in modest quantities in juice form and diluted with water.
- To alleviate gas, drink peppermint or chamomile tea; change your position or try gentle movement.
- Heat, such as from a hot water bottle, may help, as may bending over, lying on your stomach, or lying on your back with knees bent and a pillow over your abdomen.
- If stress is a factor, try relaxation exercises (explained in "Anxiety and Fear") or listening to relaxing music.

Homeopathic Remedies

Allopathic medicines such as antacids attempt to soothe symptoms by decreasing the acid of the stomach or the hypermotility of the gut. But this can weaken the body and hamper your ability to cure yourself: reducing the acid weakens the ability of the stomach to digest food, and reducing hypermotility limits the body's attempt to quickly remove the irritant from the gut. Homeopathy helps by strengthening the stomach lining to withstand irritants and by increasing the efficacy of the crampy gut activity, diarrhea or vomiting can go away sooner. The most commonly used homeopathic remedies for this condition are:

- Nux vomica. For heartburn, nausea, and burping caused by overindulgence in alcohol, tobacco, coffee, food, mental stimulation; when headache and irritability are present and the person cannot bear noise, odor, or light; when the person is in the habit of using allopathic medicines for indigestion. Nux is the "hangover medicine" for a sour or heavy stomach the morning after.
- Arsenicum. When abdominal pain or indigestion is accompanied by violent vomiting, painful diarrhea, severe nausea, and severe chills; the person is exhausted, weak, and fearful; there is severe thirst but the person drinks only small sips; symptoms are worse at night, especially around midnight, and the person cannot bear the sight or smell of food. Arsenicum is particularly useful when symptoms are due to food

poisoning, the ill effects of melons, watery fruits, or vegetables.

- Ipecac. For severe persistent nausea and vomiting; when vomiting does not relieve nausea; vomit contains mucus; abdominal pains are "pinching" or sharp and accompanied by a lot of gas; there is diarrhea; when symptoms are made worse by the smell of food or after eating or drinking.

- Pulsatilla. When indigestion follows overeating of rich, fatty foods and symptoms include bloating and a heavy feeling; the person is not thirsty and craves open air.

- Colocynthis. This works best when pains are cramplike and the person doubles over or presses the painful area for relief; the pain may or may not be accompanied by vomiting or diarrhea; when there is a strong emotional component; if eating or drinking worsens symptoms and warmth improves them.

- Magnesia phosphorica. Also useful for conditions similar to colocynthis, except warmth provides more relief than pressure, and vomiting and diarrhea are seldom present. The person is thirsty for cold drinks, has gas with belching that gives no relief, and is flatulent.

- Belladonna. When symptoms appear suddenly and include fever, nausea, vomiting, diarrhea; for sharp pains that come and go; when pain is worsened by drinking, motion, standing, and gentle pressure, and is improved with firm pressure.

- Phosphorus. This remedy also helps gastroenteritis, especially if vomiting occurs after drinking even small amounts of water; the abdomen may feel empty, which may prevent sleep.

• Bryonia. This is indicated for gastroenteritis; when the slightest movement of any part of the body can trigger symptoms including abdominal pain, nausea, vomiting, and diarrhea; when pain is relieved by pressure, lying on the affected area, or a bowel movement. The person is thirsty and drinks whole glasses of liquids.

Dosage

Choose the remedy from the above list that most closely matches your symptoms. Administer, following the Rule of Three (page 55). If after eight to twelve hours you are still experiencing abdominal pain or indigestion, repeat the same process with the next homeopathic remedy that most closely corresponds with your symptoms.

Important Precautions

If you are presently taking allopathic drugs, or are under medical treatment for a specific medical condition, it is essential to consult your homeopath or allopathic doctor before administering homeopathic remedies. Medical care should also be sought if the pain is severe, or begins near the navel and then moves to the lower right abdomen (a possible sign of appendicitis); if the pain is severely disabling; if the vomiting or diarrhea is persistent or contains blood; or if there is a possibility of poisoning.

ACNE

Most people consider acne to be the bane of adolescence, but it can also happen to adults, even those who went through their teens blemish free. Homeopathy regards teen acne differently from adult acne. In teenagers, acne may plague otherwise healthy kids; it is just one of the many changes the body undergoes during the hormonal transition of puberty. Unless it is severe, teen acne is considered normal (but treatable). However, adult acne is not part of a normal process of change, and therefore is considered to be a sign of underlying chronic illness.

The signs of acne—red, inflamed pimples, whiteheads, blackheads—occur when oil glands produce too much or dysfunctional oil (sebum). Bacteria on the skin interact with the sebum and cause abscesses to form—inflammation and plugging up of the hair follicles near the glands. Infection may set in, which can eventually cause scars.

Allopathic medicine commonly throws antibiotics at pimples—both taken internally and applied directly to the skin. Although they do kill bacteria and seem to improve the condition, antibiotics are taken for years and only serve to drive the condition deeper. Homeopathy considers acne to be the body's attempt to heal an underlying disease, so if it is suppressed the disease process shows up later as something else—depending on the person, this may be anything from depression, to menstrual disorders, to a cough. Antibiotics also upset the balance of our normal bacteria in the skin and elsewhere. Newer treatments, such as retinoic acid, also fail to get to the heart of the problem.

If you have mild acne with only a few intermittent

THE A-TO-Z GUIDE TO . . . TREATMENT

eruptions, follow the suggestions under general homeopathic care and try one of the homeopathic remedies. Severe cases require the professional homeopathic prescription of a constitutional cure. Unfortunately, even choosing the correct medicine will not clear up acne overnight. So if you get a zit the day before the prom or a big job interview, all you can do is cover it up.

General Homeopathic Home Care

- Acne is often exacerbated by allopathic drugs such as oral contraceptives or corticosteroids; talk to your doctor about stopping them or reduce the dosage if possible.
- Stress may be a factor, so try the relaxation therapies explained in "Anxiety and Fear."
- Keep skin clean, but overenthusiastic scrubbing may actually worsen acne. Avoid squeezing pimples, since this can spread infection and injure delicate, inflamed tissues. Mild astringents like witch hazel (diluted 1:1 with water) can be soothing when used daily.
- A good diet consisting of plenty of fruits and vegetables improves health generally. Chocolate and fatty foods are no longer thought to be linked to acne flare-ups.

Homeopathic Remedies

The following are most often used for treating acne:

- Calcarea sulphurica. The most successful remedy for acne; it heals infected abscesses that are discharging pus.

- Hepar sulphuris. Best for acne that is exceedingly painful and sensitive to the touch; when pimples are inflamed, and before the abscess has opened.
- Silica. For acne that easily becomes infected or when the individual pimples last a long time, or drain a long time.
- Natrum muriaticum. For skin that is even more greasy than is usual in people prone to acne.
- Nux vomica. For acne in young people, especially if the person craves spices, stimulants, and drugs, and is chilly in the morning.

Dosage

Choose the remedy from the above list that most closely matches your symptoms. Calcarea sulphurica is usually the most effective and works about 50 to 60 percent of the time. Begin with 6x potency twice a day. Because this condition is slow to go away, even when part of the normal hormonal changes of adolescence, it takes longer to treat than other acute conditions. Therefore, you will need to continue treatment for four to eight weeks. If you notice improvement, continue for three more months and then stop. If there is a relapse, try a higher potency—9 or 12c. If Calcarea is not the right medicine for the case, repeat the same process with the next homeopathic medicine that most closely corresponds with your symptoms, or see an experienced homeopath.

Important Precautions

If you are presently taking allopathic drugs, or are under medical treatment for a specific medical condition, it is essential to consult your homeopath or allopathic doctor before administering homeopathic remedies. Medical care should also be sought if the condition is severe; or if the following signs appear in an adult: general illness such as weight change, change in hair distribution, change in the menstrual cycle, change in general energy or body temperature.

ALLERGIES

Allergies are reactions of the immune system to something in your environment. A healthy immune system recognizes and destroys potentially harmful foreign infectious invaders such as bacteria and viruses, or noninfectious irritants such as pollen, dust, or animal dander.

The immune system of the allergic person works properly, it just works too hard. The trouble is that the tissue barriers are weak and let the irritant (allergen) penetrate too deeply. A violent response, such as sneezing, tearing, and inflammation, is required to expel or detoxify the allergen. As the allergic person reacts more strongly than usual to allergens such as pollen, certain foods, animal dander, molds, medicines, or chemicals, many body systems may suffer from symptoms. However, the nose, sinuses, throat, and other parts of the respiratory tract, as well as the skin and digestive system, are especially vulnerable. Allopathic medicine suppresses allergic symptoms with antihistamines, decongestants, and steroids. Such treatment stops the body's healthy, though uncomfortable, reaction to the overpenetration of irritants and leads to a deeper disease in the long run. The goal in homeopathy is to strengthen tissue barriers (nose, skin, lung, digestive tract) and strengthen the person in general.

Complete cure for recurrent or chronic allergies requires constitutional treatment by a professional homeopath. However, acute attacks may be treated in the home to alleviate symptoms without driving the disease deeper. Prevention is based on avoiding the offending substances as much as possible. There is also some evidence that breast-fed babies develop fewer allergies than bottle-fed infants.

Allergies covered in this section are contact dermatitis (skin rash), eczema, hives, and upper-respiratory-tract allergy (hay fever). See also the separate section on "Asthma," which has a variety of possible causes, including allergic reaction.

General Homeopathic Home Care

General treatment in all allergies is designed to help support barrier tissue strength and healing. Take 2 to 3 grams (2,000 to 3,000 milligrams) of vitamin C and 25,000 IU of vitamin A or beta-carotene per day in divided doses for no more than three months, drink plenty of water (two quarts per day), and rest as much as possible.

CONTACT DERMATITIS (SKIN RASH)

The list of substances that may cause this itchy skin condition is a long one. It includes plants such as poison ivy, oak, or sumac; jewelry; rubber; cosmetics and lotions; and laundry detergent residue in clothing, sheets, and towels. Diaper rash is a form of contact dermatitis that may be linked with exposure to detergent or other irritants, or to urine itself. Remember, the rash is the innate health of the body trying to detoxify the skin through inflammation. (See also "Diaper Rash" if a skin reaction affects the diapered area of an infant.)

General Homeopathic Home Care

- Try to determine the cause of the rash so you can avoid exposure to it.
- To prevent infection with bacteria or fungus, wash the rash gently with mild soap (such as Calendula soap) and water twice a day.
- Apply lotion to soothe the raw skin; wet comfrey tea compresses are particularly soothing for poison oak.
- Change clothes once or twice a day to keep the skin clean; or you may cover the affected areas with loose sterile gauze dressings.

Homeopathic Remedies

Homeopathic remedies relieve the itchiness and accelerate healing. The most often used are:

- Urtica urens. This remedy can sometimes ease the whole process if taken when the rash is just emerging, is red and itchy, but does not yet include vesicles.
- Rhus toxicodendron (poison ivy) and rhus diversiloba (poison oak). For treating rashes caused

by these plants; for other rashes that burn and itch, with blisters and inflammation; when the person is irritable and restless; symptoms are worse from scratching, exposure to open air, and at night; they are better from immersion in very hot water.

- Graphites. When skin oozes golden-colored fluid.
- Sulphur. For any type of rash when the person matches the general characteristics of the medicine listed in the Glossary of Homeopathic Remedies.
- Calendula tincture. To be applied when symptoms have begun to subside; speeds healing of raw, blistered skin. Dilute 10 drops of tincture with 1/2 cup water; apply with cotton ball four to five times a day, or use as a wet dressing. You may also apply Calendula ointment several times a day.

Dosage

Choose the remedy from the above list that most closely matches your symptoms. Administer, following the Rule of Three (page 55). If there is no improvement, proceed to the next recommended homeopathic medicine and repeat the process.

Important Precautions

If you are presently taking allopathic drugs, or are under medical treatment for a specific medical condition, it is essential to consult your homeopath or allopathic doctor before administering homeopathic medicines. If you see signs of infection such as pus and worsening inflammation, turn to the section on "Impetigo" or consult a professional.

ECZEMA

Eczema is a rash that turns the skin red and causes inflammation, itching, skin thickening, and bumps and blisters that may be dry or wet. It may arise from numerous skin conditions, but is usually equated with a particular allergic skin disorder called "atopic dermatitis." This form of eczema is a chronic condition that homeopaths believe begins in infancy. The child may eventually grow out of it, or it may continue into adulthood. Eczema can be triggered by a wide variety of substances similar to those that cause hives. Extremes of temperature and humidity, sweating, and psychological stress also appear to cause flare-ups.

Allopathy treats eczema with cortisone creams that palliate temporarily but do not cure; they have harmful immediate effects and can lead to more serious problems. Conventional medicine recognizes that cortisone cream can cause a variety of local skin reactions and irritations; it eventually thins the skin and weakens it. Contrary to popular belief, the cortisone in such creams can be absorbed through the skin: their longtime use on large areas of eczema has been found to interfere with the growth of children. Therefore, it is likely that something more subtle may occur when smaller amounts are absorbed in anyone. In addition, allopathic treatment suppresses the symptom. Some homeopaths believe it is no mere coincidence that children with eczema also tend to have asthma—suppressing the skin condition causes lung problems later on. Chronic eczema is curable when treated with constitutional medicine by a skilled homeopath, and the earlier the better.

Remember, any chronic itch, like pain, is a signal. It may be telling you that it is time to look around for irritants that are triggering the skin reaction. Each itch can have a physical irritant as well as a symbolic psychosocial meaning that helps us explore our world and understand our relationship to it. The allergic person often experiences life as a war, an assault on the body. A healing occurs when we alter that dynamic, by enhancing our barrier-tissue strength and finding our internal "safe haven."

Acute eczema is a delayed allergy reaction and can be treated safely in the home. However, acute eczema is relatively rare.

General Homeopathic Home Care

- Keep the affected areas away from water as much as possible. You may need to reduce bathing and washing, and wear protective rubber gloves for hand-washing of clothes or dishes.
- Avoid strong soaps. Use gentle soaps, without perfumes or chemicals, sparingly.
- Lubricate the skin with unscented cream or lotion.
- Try to determine and avoid triggers such as certain foods, detergents, wool clothing, and emotional stress.
- Try not to scratch, because it irritates already inflamed skin.
- Apply dressings to areas that are raw or ooze. Use gauze with wraparound dressing, if possible, to avoid the irritation of Band-Aid adhesives.

Homeopathic Remedies

The most commonly used homeopathic remedies for treating acute eczema are:

- Graphites. When the eczema is "wet," and exudes a fluid resembling honey, especially if it occurs in the flexion points (such as elbows) or on the palms of the hands, between toes, and around the genitals and mouth; symptoms worsen with warmth and around menstruation; they improve with cold applications.
- Petroleum. For dry, scaly eczema that appears during cold weather or wintertime. Symptoms are worse in winter, and from damp and cold; they are better in summer, and from dry warmth.
- Natrum muriaticum. For dry flaky crusts in elbow creases, behind the ears, and near the hairline; for oily rashes on hairy parts of the body; when the rash gets worse from warmth and better with cool weather and cold water.
- Calcarea carbonica. In infants with white or light yellow crusting skin on the scalp; when symptoms get worse from cold and better with dry warmth. Calcarea is also useful for eczema in children who have difficulty teething, and for rashes that appear on the legs, around the navel, and at flexion points such as elbows.
- Sulphur. For dry, scaly, itchy, burning eczema of the scalp; symptoms are worse with scratching or moist warmth such as bathing; better with dry warmth.

- Arsenicum. For small dry, scaly, and itchy patches that leave a red, watery skin surface.

Graphites is available in an ointment as well as an oral form. You may use this or Calendula ointment.

Dosage

Choose the medicine from the above list that most closely matches the person's symptoms. Administer according to the Rule of Three (page 55). If there is no clear response to the remedy, repeat the process with the next homeopathic remedy that most closely corresponds to the person's symptoms.

Important Precautions

If the person is presently taking allopathic drugs, or is under medical treatment for a specific medical condition, it is essential to consult a homeopath or allopathic doctor before administering homeopathic medicines. If the acute eczema returns again and again, it is probably a chronic condition and should be treated professionally.

HIVES

Hives are large red inflamed swellings ("welts") that may suddenly appear anywhere on the skin. Hives may also erupt in the respiratory passages. The welts are intensely itchy and may spread quickly, sometimes running together to create larger patches of raised angry skin. There is no crust or vesicle production, only smooth red swellings.

Their appearance is usually tied to certain foods (fruits, nuts, eggs, certain shellfish), a recent systemic streptococcal or viral infection, or other factors including medicines, insect bites, cold, and emotional stress. Sometimes the cause is never found. Acute hives may last only a few hours, a day, or a week, and so are self-limiting. Hives may also be a symptom of a chronic condition, which requires treatment by a professional homeopath.

General Homeopathic Home Care

- Some hives can be soothed with a cool, damp cloth; others grow worse with cold application.

Homeopathic Remedies

For acute isolated cases of hives, choose among these remedies:

- Apis mellifica. When symptoms arrive suddenly and welts are red; violent stinging, itching, and burning; when symptoms are worse with heat, touch, or pressure, and better with local application of cold.
- Urtica urens. This is used as an antidote to allergic reaction to shellfish; it is most effective when the itching burns and is severe; when symptoms are worse with local application of cold, or from general warmth or strenuous exercise.
- Rhus toxicodendron. For hives caused by cold weather, rubbing, wetness or perspiration.
- Dulcamara. For hives that come on at night,

especially cool nights with heavy dew, or
when weather changes from warm to cool and
damp. For hives that accompany stomach disorders.

- Pulsatilla. Think of Pulsatilla if the rash is always changing location, especially if it feels better in open air and from the cold, and is worse in
the evening and at night.

Dosage

Apis is the most commonly used homeopathic remedy
for hives and is generally indicated when the person
does not closely fit the symptom patterns for the other
remedies. Administer in the 30c potency following the
Rule of Three (page 55). Stop the medication when you
see improvement. If Apis does not bring relief, repeat
the same process with the next homeopathic medicine
that most closely corresponds with your symptoms.

Important Precautions

If the person is presently taking allopathic drugs, or is
under medical treatment for a specific medical condition, it is essential to consult a homeopath or allopathic
doctor before administering homeopathic medicines.
Also consult a physician if there is severe swelling, or if
hives appear on the mouth or tongue, or if the person
has trouble breathing. Hives that last for more than a
month may indicate internal disease and require professional evaluation.

UPPER-RESPIRATORY-TRACT ALLERGY (HAY FEVER)

The nose, throat, and eyes are often targets for airborne allergens; as a result of exposure, you sneeze (sometimes intensely and uncontrollably), your nose and eyes run and are unbearably itchy, or your nose may be stuffy; sometimes even the roof of your mouth or your ears itch too.

In many people, the problem stems from high levels of pollen—tiny grains released by plants, trees, and grasses—and so is confined to certain times of the year. Such "hay fever" usually occurs in the late summer or fall and the spring; but this depends on the geographical location and climate patterns. Dust, molds, and animal dander (from live pets or feather bedding) are also frequent upper-respiratory allergens.

Conventional medicine has improved in its treatment of hay fever; the new antihistamines do not cause the drowsiness of the older drugs, but they still have side effects and their suppression of the body's defense mechanisms, which expel the irritants, drives the condition deeper. Desensitizing injections—in which tiny amounts of allergens are used to gradually build up a tolerance—have had some success, but do not cure the underlying allergic condition. Since these allergies are chronic, only homeopathy truly offers a cure—but this requires a skilled homeopath. Treatment usually begins in the winter and generally requires two years or more. During this time, even though symptoms may still appear, no allopathic antiallergy medicines may be taken. However, homeopathic medicines that palliate symptoms may be allowed under a homeopath's guidance.

General Homeopathic Home Care

- Try to avoid the things that trigger hay fever, such as pollen, animal dander, or dust. Avoid heavily planted areas during hay-fever season and keep your home as dust free as possible. Use an air cleaner in bedrooms. Take up carpets and use synthetic-fiber pillows and blankets.
- Rinse your face (nose, eyes) with cool water and wash hands when you get home; wash hair frequently. These measures remove pollen and other allergens that cling to your body.
- If breathing is difficult because of swollen nasal passages, inhale water vapor from a humidifier to open them up.
- If eyes are very irritated, rinse them periodically with sterile saline solution (salt water available at drug stores) to dislodge pollen and soothe inflamed membranes.

Homeopathic Remedies

The remedies suggested here will lessen allergic symptoms during an acute attack whether you are undergoing a constitutional cure or not. They may reduce your need for allopathic medicine or eliminate it entirely. Unlike constitutional remedies, they will not prevent or reduce the intensity of future attacks.

- Allium cepa. If symptoms include a copious burning discharge from the nose, frequent sneezing, a red and sore nose, and watery eyes that are sore and burn. Allium is particularly indicated when the person sneezes upon entering a warm room. Possible accompanying symptoms include headache, cough, and hoarseness—all of which improve in the open air.

- Euphrasia. When most of the symptoms affect the eyes, which tear, swell, burn, and are sensitive to light. The discharge from the eye is irritating to the skin but nasal discharge is bland and sneezing does not occur in violent bouts. Euphrasia is also useful for asthma triggered by hay fever.

- Sabadilla. When there is a profuse, watery nasal discharge, frequent and sudden bursts of sneezing, an itchy nose, and red watery eyes are accompanied by an urge to swallow frequently; symptoms may be either better or worse outdoors in the open air. Useful for asthma from hay fever.

- Nux vomica. For hay fever characterized by a stuffy nose, especially at night and outdoors. There is frequent or sudden bursts of sneezing, and an acrid nasal discharge in the daytime. Nux may be helpful when hay fever triggers asthma.

- Arsenicum album. When there is a thin and watery mucus that burns the upper lip, a stuffy nose, and a lot of sneezing; these symptoms are worse in the open air, and better indoors. Arsenicum is also useful for asthma triggered by hay fever.

- Pulsatilla. When the eyes produce a sticky, thick yellow discharge and eyes are itchy and burn, there is copious tearing, and eyes feel worse with warmth.

- Ambrosia (Ragweed). For eyes that water heavily and are intolerably itchy, a stuffed-up feeling in the nose and head, and watery mucus from nose with or without frequent sneezing.

• Wyetha. When symptoms include intense itching of the back of the mouth or behind the nose.

Euphrasia (Eyebright) may also be used externally to soothe itchy eyes: Get the tincture form and dilute it in sterile water (10 drops of tincture in 1/2 cup water). Use this as an eye bath three or four times a day, or make as a tea and use as a wet dressing.

Dosage

Choose the remedy from the above list that most closely matches the person's symptoms. Administer according to the Rule of Three (page 55) as needed during the hay-fever season. If there is no clear response to the medicine, repeat the process with the next homeopathic medicine that most closely corresponds to the person's symptoms.

Important Precautions

If the person is presently taking allopathic drugs, or is under medical treatment for a specific medical condition, it is essential to consult a homeopath or allopathic doctor before administering homeopathic medicines.

ANXIETY AND FEAR

Life is full of experiences that may cause some people to become temporarily fearful. Even people we consider

to be psychologically strong and healthy may be prone
to preexam jitters or preinterview nerves; a person may
fret about an upcoming wedding, giving a speech or
presentation, or performing in a concert, play, or com-
petition. In other cases, a recent unanticipated frightening experience may shake us up for a while—a near-
miss car accident or a natural disaster such as an earth-
quake, hurricane, flood, or fire.

We may become paralyzed with fear, or can't stop
shaking; we may think constantly about the future or
past event, lose sleep, and be unable to concentrate,
which makes dealing with the experience more difficult.

Homeopathy can soothe both adults and children
through the emotional ill-effects of such specific crises.
Long-standing or chronic fear and free-floating anxiety,
however, are deep-seated conditions and require constitutional treatment by a professional homeopath.

General Homeopathic Home Care

- As with all symptoms, suppressing your fear is
  not healthy in the long run. Generally, it is better to acknowledge your fear and talk to another
  person or persons in a safe, supportive environment.
- Remember: emotions help you heal, and allow
  the bodymind to return to a balanced healthy
  state, so don't "beat yourself up" for feeling the
  way you do. The right amount of fear can actually help us perform better, or stimulate thinking
  about how to minimize fearful experiences in the
  future.
- The more important and deeper the feeling of

fear, the more likely that unhealed fears in the
past are being stirred up. But even this can be
helpful, because it brings up issues that are still
bothering you and should be dealt with.

• Listen to your own individual needs: Do you feel
better when you are left alone, or are in the company of others? Do you find comfort in talking
to people who share similar experiences and
feelings? Can you find ways to distract yourself
until the fear passes?

• Relaxation techniques are tools that help us con-
sciously relax for a short period every day and
can help calm fears. Exercise, yoga, meditation,
biofeedback, and massage are among the most
popular and effective ways to reach a state of
relaxation—they are like taking a minivacation.
There are many books, tapes, courses, and one-
on-one training opportunities for you to learn
relaxation techniques. Or you might want to
try progressive muscle relaxation, described below.

Progressive Muscle Relaxation. This is a simple,
no-frills technique used to relax the bodymind by
alternately tensing and relaxing the muscles. It
may take about one-half hour at first, but with
time it becomes easier and you will achieve the
relaxed state sooner. Make sure you are in quiet
surroundings—no TV or radio playing, telephone
unplugged or off the hook. Have the room temperature on the warm side; keep a blanket handy in
case you feel chilly during the process. To begin, lie
down on a comfortable surface, close your eyes,

and take a few deep, slow breaths. Direct your attention to your right leg. Stretch it away from your body, pointing your foot hard; hold until it begins to tremble slightly and then let go and allow it to relax completely. Repeat with the left leg. Next, move your attention to your right arm, stretch it, and then let it go limp as you did with your leg. Clench your hand into a tight fist; hold and then release. Stretch the fingers out straight; hold and then release. Proceed to alternately contract and then relax the muscles of your hips (contract buttocks, then release), waist (pull in your stomach, then release), back (press your lower back to the floor, then release), chest (contract your ribs inward so your chest becomes concave, then release), shoulders (scrunch them up toward your ears, then relax them back down), and scalp (wiggle your ears, move your eyebrows up and down, then release). Finally, move to your face: open your mouth and eyes wide; next, scrunch them in; and then let the muscles go. Take a few deep, slow breaths (breathe slowly and rhythmically throughout) and repeat the exercise. Then just lie still for ten minutes or so, allowing your mind to let go of whatever is bothering you. If thoughts enter your mind, just let them float by without trying to stop them. When you are ready, stretch your arms overhead, point your feet, take a deep breath, and gradually open your eyes and return to your surroundings.

Homeopathic Remedies

The remedies most often used to quiet acute fears are:

- Gelsemium. An often-used remedy for anticipatory fear before giving a speech or for preexam anxiety; when the person becomes dull with fear, can't concentrate, and his mind goes blank.
- Aconite. When the fearful person is physically and mentally restless; he may have trouble sleeping and be hypersensitive to noise, light, and touch. The person trembles, looks pale, and is full of dread.
- Ignatia. For the ill effects of worrying. The person has changeable moods and symptoms, is introspective, silent, and brooding. He may feel as though there is a lump in his throat.
- Pulsatilla. When the fear is accompanied by crying, or the anxiety causes trembling and flushing. Anxious or fearful thoughts prevent him from falling asleep or staying asleep, and he wants company and support.
- Lycopodium. Another superb remedy for people with fear about upcoming events such as public speaking, taking an exam, or any other social situation that causes them to fear what other people will think of them. The person may wake up from fright or anxious dreams.

Dosage

Choose the remedy from the above list that most closely matches your symptoms. Administer, following the Rule of Three (page 55). If the remedy does not prove to be effective, repeat the same process with the next homeopathic remedy that most closely corresponds with your symptoms.

Important Precautions

If you are presently taking allopathic drugs, or are under medical treatment for a specific medical condition, it is essential to consult your homeopath or allopathic doctor before administering homeopathic remedies. Medical care should also be sought if the symptoms of anxiety are accompanied by worsening or severe physical symptoms such as chest pain, abdominal pain, headache, difficulty breathing, or any other dramatic change in ability to function.

ASTHMA

Asthma is a chronic condition that causes episodes of wheezing and shortness of breath. The throat and chest feel tight, the person may cough and produce thick phlegm. Symptoms of asthma range from mild to severe, and may come on suddenly and dramatically, or gradually worsen with increasing difficulty breathing. An attack may be as brief as five minutes or last for days on end.

During a particularly severe attack, the person feels as if he is suffocating; wheezing may be heard all the way across the room; and he may have a rapid pulse and sweat profusely. The symptoms are due to a temporary contraction in the muscles of the breathing passages, which swell and fill with mucus.

Asthma is quite frightening and may cause death;

sometimes it is so severe that allopathic drugs are appropriate and necessary, in spite of homeopathic treatment. Commonly used drugs include ephedrine and steroids to relax the muscles of the constricted passageways, inhalers, and expectorants to clear the phlegm. These all have side effects and when used frequently or improperly, they can lose their effectiveness and cause a person to be dependent on them.

A professional homeopath can provide constitutional medicines that reduce the frequency and severity of this chronic, deep, and often genetically determined condition. Homeopathic home care and remedies may palliate the symptoms of an attack, but be sure to have the disease diagnosed professionally and understand your particular symptom pattern before attempting to treat asthma yourself. And consult with your doctor before administering any self-remedy.

There are three types of asthma. *Allergic asthma* results when the person is extremely hypersensitive to minimal amounts of allergens or mild irritants in the environment. These include pollen, dust, animal dander, feather pillows, certain foods, smoke, and auto exhaust. The person with allergic asthma often has a long history of allergies, beginning in childhood, and a general tendency toward allergies usually runs in the family. Some develop allergic asthma as children; others develop it later in life.

Reactive asthma is also stimulated by an irritant, but the irritant must be present in more than a minimal amount. Common irritants include bacteria related to severe upper-respiratory infections, bronchitis, and pneumonia; some people suffer asthmatic attacks every time they get sick. Another trigger is emphysema or other noninfectious lung disease. Sometimes an overwhelming amount of dust, such as occurs in a dust storm or in certain occupations, can also cause a reactive asthma attack. In some people, fatigue, hormonal changes, exercise, and changes in the temperature or humidity can aggravate an attack.

Finally, there is *psychogenic asthma*—instead of a physical cause, it has an emotional trigger. The person prone to this type of asthma is expressing his or her emotions on a physical level.

General Homeopathic Home Care

- Breathing exercises such as yoga-type abdominal and abdominal and chest breathing are very helpful between attacks. In addition, regular vigorous exercise between attacks helps strengthen the lungs.
- Relaxation exercises are helpful for daily self-care and can be used at the onset of an attack to lessen symptoms. See the section on "Anxiety and Fear" for more information about relaxation techniques.
- Drinking plenty of fluids helps loosen mucus and replace the water your body loses during the shallow, rapid breathing and increased perspiration during an asthma attack.

Homeopathic Remedies

The most common homeopathic remedies for acute asthma attacks are:

- Arsenicum. When there is marked fearfulness, restlessness, and weakness, Arsenicum is the

most useful remedy. Symptoms are worse between midnight and 3:00 A.M. and there may be
coughing or hay-fever symptoms; people who
respond to Arsenicum tend to feel chilly and be
thirsty for frequent small sips.

- Pulsatilla. For asthma attacks that bring about
phlegm that causes the person to cough; wheezing is worse in the evening and at night and
symptoms are worse after eating. Pulsatilla is
recommended for people who are sweet, affectionate, and clinging, are generally uncomfortable in warm rooms, and are not thirsty,
regardless of the specific asthma symptoms.

- Ipecac. When there is a lot of phlegm and symptoms such as wheezing come in intense spasms.
You can often hear the phlegm rattle as the person breathes or coughs; coughing is intense, and
may bring up food or mucus. The person is pale
and weak and nausea usually accompanies the
respiratory symptoms.

- Spongia. In asthma that is of the dry variety,
with little or no phlegm; noisy, labored breathing and a "barking" cough may be present; attacks are precipitated by a cold or a chill; the
wheezing is worse after sleep, and the shortness
of breath is made worse by lying down and
movement.

Dosage

Choose the homeopathic remedy from the above list
that most closely matches the person's symptoms. Administer using the Rule of Three (page 55). Stop the
medicine when you notice real improvement. If there is

no improvement with the remedy of choice, you may repeat the dose anyway. You may also repeat the remedy if symptoms respond initially and then return, but not more than once every two hours, or ten times in two days. If there is no response at all or symptoms are severe, get professional advice.

Important Precautions

Asthma can be a life-threatening disease. Call your physician if the attack causes severe shortness of breath, if the person has a bad sore throat and has difficulty swallowing, or if a child is wheezing and drooling heavily. You should also consult a physician if this attack seems different from past experiences, if a child under two years of age is wheezing, or if the person cannot comfortably walk around the house or talk because of shortness of breath. As is the case with all conditions, if the person is presently taking allopathic drugs, or is under medical treatment for a specific medical condition, it is essential to consult a homeopath or allopathic doctor before administering homeopathic medicines.

BACK AND NECK PROBLEMS

Backache is one of the most common complaints of modern civilization—80 percent of American adults suffer from back pain at some point in their lives, and it is the leading cause of worker disability. It is also one of the most difficult and frustrating conditions to treat allopathically—treatment consists of painkillers, muscle relaxers, antidepressants, and surgery.

Your "backbone" or spine consists of *vertebrae*

stacked one on top of the other, ending with the *sacrum* (five vertebrae that fuse together during childhood) and then the *coccyx* (three or four small vertebrae that fuse during our twenties). In between the vertebrae are spongy *disks* that cushion the vertebral surfaces and allow the back to bend without injuring the spinal cord running through the column of vertebrae. Surrounding the spinal column are muscles, ligaments, and nerves, all in a complex interrelated pattern that works together to support most of our body weight while allowing us to move freely.

Most people who suffer from backaches never pinpoint the exact cause. It may be a specific injury due to overexertion or sudden movement; or it could be a lifelong posture problem finally catching up with you; or it might occur after staying in an unusual or uncomfortable position for a prolonged period of time.

Often a muscle strain is involved. Ligaments along the spine, and muscles in the abdomen and lower back, keep the back in balance. When these muscles are weak, they can't support the torso properly. As a result, they can overstretch and then strongly contract, giving us a painful muscle spasm. Being out of shape is part of the problem, and being overweight compounds the precarious situation. Ligaments (tough bands that attach bones to nearby bones) can become overstretched due to years of poor posture, putting more strain on the muscles, and allowing joints to wear out, both of which can add to back problems. Emotions influence our muscles and back as well. Back complaints can even be "solutions" to hidden social and emotional conflicts or misunderstandings.

We experience back problems in five main areas: going from the top down, they are:

- *Stiff (or "wry") neck (torticollis),* which often occurs spontaneously for unknown reasons; it may be related to holding the neck in an unnatural position for a long time—as when one cradles a phone between ear and shoulder—or to emotional tension.
- *Lower back pain,* which occurs behind the waist and is often related to overexertion, overlifting, sitting on the ground for a long time, or sleeping on the ground or a soft bed.
- *Sacroiliac sprain,* which occurs below the waist and behind the hips; it is usually related to overlifting and sometimes to imbalanced posture, such as carrying a child on your hip.
- *Coccyx injury,* in which the "tailbone" is bruised in a fall.
- *Sciatica,* in which sharp pain shoots down the back of the leg; it is related to muscle spasms, joint strains, and in some people to deterioration or injury of a disk between the vertebrae, which irritates the nerve (herniated disk).

General Homeopathic Home Care

Homeopathic remedies can speed healing of acute back pain due to injury, but other healing systems can contribute as well, such as acupuncture, chiropractic, osteopathy, massage, and physical therapy. In addition, the following will help heal and/or minimize back problems:

- Apply wet heat to ease the pain. Never use dry heat directly on the skin, as it can dehydrate the tissues.

- You may need to rest the injury for a day or two, but prolonged bed rest is not advisable. Use the time of rest to think about conflicts and emotions that may be contributing to your backache, especially when no severe injury is involved.
- Begin a program of back-strengthening exercises and make sure you warm up before and cool down after you exercise.
- Learn the proper way to use your back, especially when lifting heavy objects: bend from the knees, not from the waist, and use your thigh muscles, not your back muscles. Avoid lifting until your back is healed.
- A physical therapist, chiropractor, or osteopath can teach you how to move, stand, sit, sleep, bend, turn, and reach properly to reduce the stress on your back and help forestall future problems. There are also videotapes and "back schools" or "back clinics" that teach good body mechanics.
- Change positions as often as possible. If you have a sedentary job or life, sit less often—sitting puts a strain on your lower back. Lie down to read, stand to talk on the phone, and shift positions and take frequent breaks (about every hour) to move your back. Spending long hours standing also stresses the back.
- Use a back support when sitting, such as a "lumbar roll" or pillow, or a rolled-up towel taped securely to the chair back.
- Lose weight if you are overweight.

Homeopathic Remedies

The homeopathic remedies most often used for back problems are:

- Arnica. For pain that feels like a bruise and is provoked by exercise or lifting a heavy object improperly. Arnica is especially useful as the first remedy after an injury or strain.
- Hypericum. For lower back pain due to a direct blow to the spine, or if there are shooting pains. Hypericum is especially useful for the initial treatment of a coccyx injury and is often followed by treatment with Silica.
- Rhus toxicodendron. For pain in the neck or lower back that is accompanied by stiffness; symptoms are worse with initial motion or cold, wet weather, and better with continual motion and application of heat. Rhus tox is one of the best sciatica remedies. If Rhus tox seems to be indicated, but doesn't work completely, try Calcarea florica.
- Bryonia. For pain in the lower back; symptoms are worse with slight movement, and during the menstrual period. This is a good sciatica remedy.
- Pulsatilla. For aching, pressing pain in the lower back or small of the back; when the back feels weak and tired and getting up is difficult; useful for sciatica. Symptoms are worse before or during the menstrual period or with initial movement; they are better with gentle continuous exercise such as slow walking.
- Lycopodium. For lower back pain accompanied by stiffness and caused by lifting; symptoms are

worse during initial movement and while getting
up from sitting; better after passing wind, urinating, or movement. Sciatica is worse from sitting and from pressure.

- Silica. For back pain after a fall or manual labor;
the back feels sore, bruised, stiff, and weak; pain
is worse from sitting and at night. Silica is especially useful after using Hypericum for an injured coccyx.

- Calcarea carbonica. For pain in the lower back;
if there is an aching, sprained feeling; pain is related to lifting.

- Phosphorus. For pain in the lower back or between shoulder blades, and the pain feels better
when it is massaged. In sciatica Phosphorus is
especially useful if there is burning pain that
worsens while lying on the painful side.

Dosage

Choose the remedy from the above list that most
closely matches your symptoms. Administer, following
the Rule of Three (page 55). If the medicine does not
prove to be effective, repeat the same process with the
next homeopathic medicine that most closely corresponds with your symptoms.

Important Precautions

If you are presently taking allopathic drugs, or are under medical treatment for a specific medical condition,
it is essential to consult your homeopath or allopathic
doctor before administering homeopathic medicines.
Seek medical attention if the back pain is accompanied

by fever, if you have trouble with either your bowels or your bladder, your urine smells unusual or has blood in it, or you have difficulty moving or feeling your legs. Back pain can be an indication of serious health problems such as arthritis, kidney disease, or cancer. Recurrent back pain or pain that doesn't improve within one week of homeopathic treatment should also be evaluated professionally.

BEDWETTING (ENURESIS)

This is usually a problem of childhood, but the tendency can persist into adolescence, and even into adulthood. Some nighttime "accidents" are to be expected among children up to age six or so, as the ability to control the bladder at night is more difficult to learn than control during the day.

No one knows why some children wet their beds. One theory is that wetters are very deep sleepers who have a smaller-than-usual bladder, or an overly sensitive bladder that feels an uncontrollably strong urge to empty. Heredity may be a factor. Or for some reason, the brain does not learn or remember its role in the delicate interplay that must occur between the urinary system and other systems that control the bladder. Sometimes food allergies or sensitivities promote bladder problems: milk, citrus fruits, chocolate, and sugar have been most often singled out. And sometimes the emotions come into play, as a variety of stresses seem to worsen or trigger bedwetting, or cause it to return in a child who has been dry for some time. Rarely, an identifiable physical abnormality is the culprit.

Enuresis usually resolves itself naturally, but persistent problems are cause for concern, and a source of embarrassment and inconvenience for children and adults alike. Once a bladder infection or structural abnormality has been ruled out, there are a number of conventional approaches used to treat enuresis. These include hypnosis, behavior modification, waking the child up during the night, using a "wetness alarm" device, and certain medications. Homeopathically, a constitutional remedy may help. If your child is otherwise healthy, you may try the homeopathic medicines listed here.

General Homeopathic Home Care

- Since bedwetting usually disappears as the child matures, the most important thing you can do is to provide a guilt-free, loving, and reassuring environment as you wait for nature to take its course. Avoid putting psychological pressure on the child, which could actually make things worse.
- Try to discover if there are emotional stresses involved, such as family troubles, troubles at school, the birth of a sibling, or moving to a new home.
- If you suspect food allergy or sensitivity, try eliminating prime suspects one at a time to see if there is any improvement.
- Restricting the amount of fluid a child drinks close to bedtime usually has no impact; however, waking the child during the night to urinate in the bathroom sometimes meets with success.

Homeopathic Remedies

The homeopathic remedies commonly used for bedwetting are:

- Sepia. Used for children who wet the bed early in the evening, especially girls who dislike attention and sympathy.
- Rhus toxicodendron. This remedy is especially useful for boys.
- Pulsatilla. When the child is weepy, gentle, sensitive, and tends to sleep with her hands above her head; the symptom is worse when the room is warm and stuffy.
- Causticum. This is useful for children who wet soon after falling asleep, and for whom the problem is worse in winter and cold weather, and better in summer. There may also be some dribbling during the day when the child coughs or sneezes.

Dosage

Choose the remedy from the above list that most closely matches the symptoms. Administer one single dose before bed for three nights in a row and wait for four weeks to gauge if there has been any improvement. If there is, repeat the medicine and wait another four weeks. If there is no noticeable improvement, try the next medicine that most closely resembles your child's symptom picture or see a homeopath for this condition.

Important Precautions

If your child is presently taking allopathic drugs, or is under medical treatment for a specific medical condition, it is essential to consult your homeopath or allopathic doctor before administering homeopathic medicines. Medical care should also be sought if your child has any other symptoms that indicate a bladder infection: frequent or painful urination, blood in the urine, abdominal pain, or fever. Children over six years old who still wet the bed frequently should also be evaluated by a professional, as should a dry child who suddenly starts to wet again.

BLADDER INFECTIONS (CYSTITIS)

Bladder infections can occur in anyone—men, women, and children. However, women are affected most often (ten times as often as men) and about 15 percent of women experience repeated bouts of cystitis throughout their lives. Although you may have an infection without noticeable symptoms, most people do suffer from at least one of the following telltale signs: burning sensation during urination, a strong urge to urinate even when little urine is passed, frequent urination (often of small amounts), a cramping feeling, and itching. Some people also have cloudy or blood-tinged urine, lower abdominal or back pain, fever, nausea, vomiting, chills, and a general malaise.

As with all infections, cystitis results from the combination of the person's weakened resistance to infection and the presence of "germs"—in this case bacteria. In women, bacteria from the anus of the digestive tract don't have far to go to reach the urethra (the tube leading from the bladder to the outside of the body). Women's urethras are only one-half inch long (compared to men's, which are several inches long and located some distance from the anus), so bacteria have only a short trip to the bladder. If the area has been irritated, for example by physical sex, bike riding, or the inflammation caused by a vaginal infection, a woman's ability to resist a bladder infection may be weakened.

Cystitis may progress to the kidneys or bloodstream, potentially serious conditions, so it should be diagnosed initially by a health professional, and monitored if symptoms are severe, prolonged, or recurrent. Antibiotics may rid the body of the current crop of bacteria, but will not strengthen the body to resist future infections.

General Homeopathic Home Care

- The moment you notice symptoms, start drinking large amounts of water to help your bladder flush out bacteria. Cranberry juice and vitamin C supplements are thought to slow the growth of bacteria.

To prevent future occurrences of cystitis:

- Make sure you always follow good hygiene—wipe from front to back after a bowel movement; change sanitary napkins and tampons frequently during your periods.
- Urinate before and after having sex; drinking a glass of water will help make this easier.
- Make sure you drink enough fluids generally

(two quarts per day) and urinate every two hours or so to regularly flush away bacteria.
- Avoid products and practices that could irritate delicate urogenital tissues, such as deodorant products, tight clothing, and caffeine. Irritation may occur from an improperly fitted diaphragm, so check the size with your health professional; if you suspect spermicidal foams and jellies may be causing an irritation, try changing brands.

Homeopathic Remedies

The remedies most often used for bladder infections are:

- Aconite. Used at the first sign of a bladder infection if the symptoms are sudden and severe.
- Cantharis. The most commonly used homeopathic remedy for this condition. The symptoms are classic: the urge to urinate is frequent, and may occur before, during, or after the bladder is emptied, as may burning, stabbing pains in the urethra. The person may be restless and frantic because of the severe pain; increased sexual desire may be present. Cantharis is the classic remedy for cystitis after sex (honeymoon cystitis).
- Nux vomica. When symptoms follow excess alcohol, coffee, certain foods, or drugs; when there is pain in the bladder during urination, or in the urethra before or during urination; there may be needlelike pains in the urethra.
- Pulsatilla. For cases where the pain is not intense, but it does burn; the urine flows in small amounts and dribbling may occur when the per-

son coughs, sneezes, or laughs. The person is not thirsty and symptoms are worse from lying on the back.

- Apis. When there is severe pain and urgency that is worse at night and with heat, but better with cold; the abdomen may be sensitive to touch and urination occurs only in dribbles despite straining.
- Mercurius. When the pain is worse when not urinating, and at night.

Dosage

Choose the remedy from the above list that most closely matches your symptoms. Administer following the Rule of Three (page 55). If the remedy does not prove to be effective, repeat the same process with the next homeopathic medicine that most closely corresponds with your symptoms.

Important Precautions

If you are presently taking allopathic drugs, or are under medical treatment for a specific medical condition, it is essential to consult your homeopath or allopathic doctor before administering homeopathic medicines. Medical care should also be sought if there is pain in the kidneys, blood in the urine, headache, fever, chills, vomiting, or nausea. People with diabetes, high blood pressure, kidney disease, or recurrent cystitis should also consult a health practitioner, as should parents of children who have symptoms of urinary-tract infection.

BOILS

A boil is a bacterial infection of the skin (it often starts in a hair follicle) that happens after the bacteria get through the protective outer layer of the skin. There may be a small wound, which children often get during normal play, or which an adult might get from shaving. Poor hygiene and general weakness are also contributing factors.

Once the bacteria enter the skin's deeper layers, the body sends healing blood to the area; the skin becomes hot, swollen, red, and can be quite painful. The nodule grows larger and pus forms—a combination of fluid from the blood, dead immune cells, and the bacteria. Boils may be only 1/4 inch wide, or grow to one or two inches. Eventually, a boil comes to a "head," which then opens up and lets the pus drain way. This usually relieves the pressure and eases the pain, and healing follows. (In some instances, the pus head does not open and drain; instead the material it contains is reabsorbed by the body.) Carbuncles are large boils with several heads and may be accompanied by fever and a general feeling of illness.

Allopathic medicine treats boils with antibiotic creams; in some cases, the nodule is surgically cut open (lanced) to encourage drainage. In recurrent cases, oral antibiotics are prescribed. By treating boils homeopathically, you can avoid all of these drastic and painful measures.

General Homeopathic Home Care

- Hot wet compresses help bring the boil to a "head"; apply twice a day for ten minutes. This

brings more blood to the area and speeds healing.
- Cover the boil with a clean gauze dressing while
it is discharging pus; once this stage is over,
leave it uncovered and exposed to the air to
heal.
- Cleanse the area frequently with soap and water.

Homeopathic Remedies

Homeopathy offers oral remedies and topical remedies
to encourage healing and build resistance to future infections. When you treat a boil in the early stages, it
disappears before pus has a chance to form. In later
stages, homeopathic remedies speed the drainage process.

- Belladonna. Best used in the early stages (within
twenty-four hours of the start of symptoms),
when the boil throbs, and is hot, red, swollen,
and painful, but there is no pus.
- Hepar sulphuricum. When the boil is very painful to even a light touch and throbs, or feels as
though a sharp splinter is in it; when it is very
sensitive to cold air. When used early, Hepar
prevents the formation of pus.
- Mercurius. Use for painful boils after pus has
formed to bring the infection to a head; when
the person is restless at night and has night
sweats; when symptoms are worse from
warmth.
- Silica. For boils that progress slowly; when the
boil is red and swollen for days without forming
pus; and when it is slow to heal even after pus

has formed and is draining. Silica is useful for lumps that remain less painful than the Hepar type, and that feel better with warmth.

- Arsenicum. Useful in both early and late stages when the boil burns and is very painful; when the person feels weak generally to a degree that is out of proportion to the condition; when the person feels chilly and restless; when the boil feels better from warmth.
- Lachesis. When the boil and skin surrounding has a blue or purple cast; when the pus is dark and thin; when the boil is sensitive to the touch.

Dosage

Choose the remedy from the above list that most closely matches your symptoms. Administer following the Rule of Three (page 55). If the medicine does not prove to be effective after twenty-four hours, repeat the same process with the next homeopathic medicine that most closely corresponds with your symptoms. You may also use Hypericum tincture (dilute 10 drops tincture in ½ cup water) as a wet dressing, which will bring the boil more quickly to a head and speed drainage.

Important Precautions

If you are presently taking allopathic drugs, or are under medical treatment for a specific medical condition, it is essential to consult your homeopath or allopathic doctor before administering homeopathic medicines. Medical care should also be sought if there is a high fever, headache, or stiff neck; if the redness or swelling is spreading from the site; if there is severe pain and lots of pus; if it doesn't heal within a week despite drainage of pus; or if the boil is on the face.

CANKER SORES AND COLD SORES

People often confuse canker sores and cold sores, and use the terms interchangeably. However, it is important to decide which condition you have, because cold sores (herpes) are contagious, while canker sores are not.

A *canker sore* is an ulcer of the mouth. The irregularly shaped sores may occur on the tongue, on the inside of the cheeks, or on the insides of the lips. Canker sores look as though the tissue has been burned, with a red ring surrounding a white circular sore. A canker sore forms when the bodymind is unable to retain the integrity of the mucous membrane lining of the mouth. This can occur from physical trauma, poor nutrition, during another illness such as an upper respiratory infection, or emotional upset.

Cold sores (also known as "fever blisters") often appear around the mouth and lips and are outward signs that the body is carrying the Type 1 herpes simplex virus. After the initial outbreak—about three to six days after infection—the herpes simplex virus normally lies dormant until there is some form of stress to throw the body off balance. The triggering stress may be physical (for example, a viral infection such as a cold, or excess sun exposure), or psychological stress. Cold sores look like tiny blisters (vesicles) in the midst of red inflamed skin. The vesicles contain a clear liquid, which may turn into pus; the vesicles open, leaving a sore, which eventually heals.

General Homeopathic Home Care

- Keep cold sores clean and dry with gentle washing with mild soap and water twice a day.
- Do not kiss other people while you have cold sores, because this can spread the herpes virus. Use separate towels until the sores are completely healed.
- Don't squeeze cold sore blisters.
- Keep sun exposure to a minimum if you have cold sores.
- To keep outbreaks of mouth sores to a minimum, avoid sunlight in excess; stay well rested; and learn to manage stress.
- Take 2 to 3 grams (2,000 to 3,000 milligrams) of vitamin C and 25,000 IU of vitamin A or beta-carotene daily, in divided doses.

Homeopathic Remedies

Mouth sores of both types respond well to both oral and topical homeopathic medications, which may be used together.

Oral Remedies

- Mercurius vivus. For *canker sores* on gums, in the mouth, and on the tongue; when pain is stinging or throbbing; when the person secretes a lot of saliva; symptoms are worse at night.
- Nux vomica. For *canker sores* when the gums are swollen, white, and bleeding.
- Sulphur. For painful, bleeding *canker sores* any-

where in the mouth; the lips are red and the gums are swollen.

- Lycopodium. For *canker sores* under the tongue; the sores may have started on the right side; symptoms are worse between 4:00 and 8:00 P.M.
- Rhus toxicodendron. For *cold sores* on lips; the sores burn and itch intensely, and symptoms include general malaise and achiness.
- Arsenicum. For *cold sores* that burn but are better when warmth is applied. Also good for *canker sores* when the pain is better from warmth, and especially when warm drinks relieve the pain.
- Natrum muriaticum. For *cold sores* in people whose symptoms accompany a fever or cold or follow disappointment or unexpressed grief; the sores are usually found around the mouth and lips, the corners of the mouth, strung like little pearls. Natrum is also useful for *canker sores* that form on the gums.

Topical Remedies

- Calendula. For cold sores apply Calendula tincture diluted 10 drops in $\frac{1}{2}$ cup of sterile water, three to four times a day, or use Calendula ointment. Canker sores may be soothed by using the same Calendula dilution as a mouthwash.
- Hypericum. Use the tincture the same way as Calendula, especially when there is tingling pain, sharp pain, or pain that shoots from the sore.

Dosage

Choose the oral remedy from the above list that most closely matches your symptoms. Administer following the Rule of Three (page 55). If the remedy does not prove to be effective, repeat the same process with the next homeopathic medicine that most closely corresponds with your symptoms.

Important Precautions

If you are presently taking allopathic drugs, or are under medical treatment for a specific medical condition, it is essential to consult your homeopath or allopathic doctor before administering homeopathic medicines. Medical care should also be sought if canker sores or cold sores recur often or are very severe, if the skin around the eyes is affected, if sores become infected, and if you see no improvement after five to seven days of homeopathic treatment. Seek immediate medical care if the eye becomes inflamed or painful.

CHICKEN POX

Chicken pox is one of the most common childhood diseases. This highly contagious viral infection causes an itchy, blisterlike rash over much of your child's body. A mild to moderate fever and upper-respiratory infection symptoms often accompany the rash.

Your child will develop a rash about two to three weeks after being exposed to the virus that causes chicken pox. Small blisters first appear on the body and scalp, and spread to the face, arms, and legs. The blisters should crust over and heal; occasionally they become infected, resulting in small sores and subsequent scars.

If sores become infected, refer to "Cuts, Scrapes, and Puncture Wounds" in the "First Aid for Injuries" section. If the fever is sudden or high, refer to "Fever" in this section.

General Homeopathic Home Care

- Keep sores clean and change your child's clothes once or twice a day.
- Help your child not scratch the sores to prevent secondary infection. Trim your child's fingernails and offer alternatives to scratching. These include showing him or her how to apply a cool compress to the sores, scratching another unaffected place on the body, and distracting with busy work or play.
- Protect sores that fester from further irritation by covering them with Band-Aids, gauze wraps, or long-sleeved cotton clothing.
- Ease your child's itch with oatmeal baths. Place one cup of quick-cooking oats in a hand towel and gather the top with a rubber band; dip in warm (not hot) bath water and pat the skin gently with the oatmeal "sponge," until the contents have dissolved into the water. Or use commercial oatmeal bath powders.
- Keep your child away from youngsters who have not had chicken pox, since it is highly contagious until the final lesions have crusted over. If your child feels well enough, it is fine to let him

or her play with other playmates who have already had chicken pox. Once you have chicken pox, you are immune to it for the rest of your life.
- Don't deliberately break the vesicles or remove an infected scab.

Homeopathic Remedies

The most common homeopathic remedies indicated for children suffering from chicken pox are:

- Rhus toxicodendron. The most highly recommended homeopathic medicine for chicken pox; for severe itching and itching that is worse from scratching; for any-size eruption and also large eruptions with pus in them; when the child feels restless generally, has insomnia, and has normal or increased thirst.
- Pulsatilla. For children who feel worse in heated conditions and more comfortable in the open air; if children cry easily; when children have a fever but little thirst.
- Antimonium tartaricum. For children in whom eruptions emerge slowly; if the eruptions are large; if, in addition to the rash, a child has a cough or bronchitis, especially if the cough is loose and produces mucus.
- Mercurius vivus. For children with offensive or profuse sweat, especially if the lesions look infected; when child feels worse at night (often with night sweats), and is intolerant to extreme heat and cold.

Preparation and Dosage

Choose the medicine from the above list that most closely matches your child's symptoms. Administer according to the Rule of Three (page 55). If after twenty-four to thirty-six hours your child has no clear response to the medicine, repeat the same process with the next homeopathic medicine that most closely corresponds with your child's symptoms, or call your health professional. If symptoms are very severe and your child is crying, restless, unable to sleep, and has a high fever, reevaluate sooner—in three to four hours.

Important Precautions

NEVER give aspirin to a child who has chicken pox. Aspirin increases the risk of a serious liver and brain illness known as Reye's syndrome. Call your pediatrician immediately if your child exhibits any of the symptoms of Reye's syndrome or encephalitis, such as vomiting, difficulty in breathing, convulsions, lack of responsiveness, or poor balance. Medical attention is also called for if skin eruptions become seriously infected, or if an infant under the age of one gets chicken pox. If you are giving your child allopathic drugs, or your child is under medical treatment for a specific medical condition, it is essential to consult your homeopath or allopathic doctor before administering homeopathic medicines.

Colds

It's not called the "common" cold for nothing—at some point just about everyone gets one, and many people get more than one cold each year. Sometimes colds, which are the body's way of dealing with viruses in our upper-respiratory tract, are only signs of our adjusting to changes in the weather. Some homeopaths feel the common cold is nature's way of telling us to slow down and take it easy—an early warning sign that we're depleting our defenses. In fact, many also hesitate to recommend medicine of any kind, even homeopathic medicine; because the condition is so benign, it's better to just rest, blow our noses, drink fluids, and let our immune systems do their job.

However, sometimes cold symptoms can be severe enough to make us truly miserable, or may drag on for days and days. In some individuals, infants and young children, for example, or the elderly, and those who are immune deficient, colds can lead to more serious problems, such as secondary bacterial infections. In these people homeopathic medicines can help—not by suppressing sniffles, a runny nose, sneezes, a fever, sore throat, or cough—but by adding support to our body's efforts to rid itself of the viral infection. Using allopathic drugs to suppress cold symptoms prolongs the illness and risks drug side-effects.

If the cold you are treating is accompanied by other symptoms, refer to other sections such as "Fever," "Coughs," and "Sore Throats."

General Homeopathic Home Care

- Make sure you take time out to rest during a cold. This doesn't necessarily mean bed rest; but do take it easy so you don't tax your reserves of energy, which could be better put to use fighting the cold.

- Drink plenty of fluids to help keep mucus flowing and replace fluid lost through sweating. Hot, bland liquids may be particularly comforting and loosen phlegm.
- Blow your nose rather than sniffling and swallowing mucus; cough up phlegm frequently. Teach young children how to do this; in infants, use a small bulb syringe to evacuate mucus from the nose.
- Avoid extreme heat, such as steam baths and saunas; and extreme cold as well.
- Take 3 to 5 grams (3,000 to 5,000 milligrams) of vitamin C per day or more in divided doses (250 milligrams for children), which some studies show can lessen the severity and duration of symptoms.
- Keep the air moist with a humidifier or vaporizer; or inhale steam from a bowl of hot water (make a hood by draping a towel over your head) to further loosen mucus and make breathing easier.
- Eat a light diet of bland, well-cooked food. The correct way of stating the old adage from American folk medicine is "If you feed a cold, you will have to starve a fever."

Homeopathic Remedies

There are a large number of homeopathic remedies useful for cold symptoms. The most commonly used are:

- Aconite. Recommended only during the early stage of a cold, especially when the cold symptoms appear suddenly and violently after exposure to cold weather or wind; when there is a clear watery runny nose, and a lot of sneezing; there may be a red, hot, sore throat, fever, and coughing; and the person may be restless and anxious, but not delirious.

- Belladonna. Also used in the earliest stage of a cold that has appeared suddenly after the person has become chilled, particularly when there is a high fever and a flushed face; the person may feel a pounding in the head and be restless, irritable, anxious, and delirious; there is a runny nose and often a dry sore throat and a cough that may be very painful.

- Ferrum phosphoricum. This is also a useful medicine for the early signs of a cold, which may be only a vague sense of not feeling quite well; for colds that occur after exposure to dampness.

- Arsenicum. For established colds in people who feel chilly, and who sneeze violently and frequently; their noses feel ticklish and irritated and produce a watery discharge that irritates and burns the upper lip; the dry, hacking cough may accompany the cold, which tends to spread to the chest. The person is thirsty for small sips of liquid, and experiences restless sleep, especially around midnight. (Arsenicum may prevent chest involvement.)

- Allium cepa. When the cold symptoms include an irritating watery nasal discharge, copious tearing of the eyes, which may also be red and burn, and strong sneezing spasms; the larynx may tickle and there may be a dry, painful cough; symptoms are worse indoors, with warmth, and in the evening; better in the open air.

- Euphrasia. Helpful if the nasal discharge is watery and bland, while tears are irritating.
- Hepar sulphuricum. For colds that appear after exposure to cold weather; the nasal discharge starts out as watery and then turns thick and yellow, smells bad, and drips down the throat; the throat feels as if there is a splinter in it and there may be spasms of coughing; the person feels chilly, yet perspires, and is sensitive to drafts, which trigger sneezing.
- Pulsatilla. Very useful for colds that have mainly nasal symptoms; mucus is thick, yellow or yellow-green, and nonirritating; it may smell bad and usually alternates with a thinner discharge; the nose may run in fresh air and in the morning, and become stuffy indoors and at night.
- Kali bichromicum. For ropy, thick nasal mucus.
- Nux vomica. For nasal congestion that is worse at night in a person who feels generally chilly.

There are many other remedies that homeopaths find beneficial in treating people with colds; if none of the above symptom pictures match or symptoms are vague, you may want to study the "Glossary of Homeopathic Remedies" and compare the following remedies' general characteristics: Natrum mur, Gelsemium, Bryonia, Phosphorus, Spongia, Sepia, and Sulphur.

Dosage

Choose the remedy from the above list that most closely matches your symptoms. Administer following the Rule of Three (page 55). If the remedy does not prove to be effective, repeat the same process with the next homeopathic remedy that most closely corresponds with your symptoms. Bear in mind that symptoms can change markedly and you may need to retake the case before choosing another remedy.

Important Precautions

If you are presently taking allopathic drugs, or are under medical treatment for a specific medical condition, it is essential to consult your homeopath or allopathic doctor before administering homeopathic medicines. Medical care should also be sought if the cold symptoms are unusually severe, or if there is severe difficulty breathing or shortness of breath, chest pain, convulsions, delirium, high fever, extreme weakness, a stiff neck, wheezing, severe headache, sudden unexpected vomiting, or if stools are light colored. Also consult your homeopath if you get colds frequently or if they are severe and long lasting.

CONJUNCTIVITIS (EYE INFLAMMATION OR PINKEYE)

Conjunctivitis is an inflammation of the thin membrane (conjunctiva) lining the eye and inner surface of the eyelids. The triggering mechanism is either a bacterium or virus (infectious conjunctivitis); or an allergy or other irritant, such as pollen, dust, smoke, smog, chemical fumes, or overexposure to glaring sunlight.

Bacterial infections generally produce a thick yellow

or yellow-green discharge; viral infections and allergies cause a thin watery discharge. In any type of conjunctivitis, the eyes may be bloodshot. The lids look red, swollen, and puffy; there may be a dry and gritty or "sandy" feeling in spite of heavy discharge or watering. Allergic conjunctivitis is generally alone in causing noticeable itching; as is the case with inflammation due to irritants, it usually occurs in both eyes simultaneously soon after exposure to the cause. Infectious conjunctivitis usually affects first one eye and then soon spreads to the other. Infectious conjunctivitis usually goes away in about ten days, without any treatment; allopathic treatment involves antibiotic eyedrops for bacterial infections, but there is no effective treatment for viral infections. Allergic conjunctivitis is treated with antihistamines, but resolves itself soon after exposure to the allergen stops. Although it is usually easy to distinguish among the various types of conjunctivitis, homeopathic evaluation and treatment hinges on the total symptom picture and pays little or no attention to the specific triggering factor.

See also "Colds," "Allergies," or refer to "Eye Injuries" in the "First Aid for Injuries" section if the conjunctivitis is related to one of those conditions.

General Homeopathic Home Care

- Bathe the affected eye in plain warm water to soothe it and rinse away the discharge.
- Maintain good hygiene and wash your hands after touching the infected eye to avoid spreading infection to the other eye or another person.

- Avoid rubbing the eye to relieve the itching; this will only irritate the eye and worsen the condition.
- For noninfectious conjunctivitis caused by an irritant or allergy, you may find rinsing with eyedrops (plain sterile saline, or salt water [a pinch of salt in 6 to 8 ounces of water], or "artificial tears") helps soothe and lubricate dry, irritated eyes.

Homeopathic Remedies

The most-often recommended remedies for conjunctivitis are:

- Belladonna. When symptoms are intense: bloodshot eyes; dry, burning conjunctiva; swollen eyelids; shooting or throbbing pain; sensitivity to light; and profuse watery tears.
- Euphrasia. Especially useful when symptoms are due to allergic reaction; symptoms include plentiful, acrid, burning tears, which may develop into a thicker discharge; a feeling of dryness or "sandiness" to the eyes; burning, red, swollen eyelids; a sensitivity to light. There may be some nasal discharge.
- Pulsatilla. For conjunctivitis characterized by profuse, thick, smelly yellow-green discharge, profuse tearing, and eyes that itch and burn. These symptoms are worse in the evening, and from warmth; better from fresh air, cold, and washing the eyes with cold water. Pulsatilla is often the medicine of choice for infants with eyes stuck shut from mucus.

- Aconite. When the key symptoms are bloodshot eyes that ache, burn, and are sensitive to light; they may feel dry and "sandy"; symptoms are worse in cold dry wind, which causes eyes to water.
- Sulphur. For eyes that burn, itch, water, are sensitive to light, and feel "sandy"; the edges of the eyelids may be sore, red, irritated, and ulcerated; eyes water more in fresh air and eyes feel worse after bathing them in water.
- Apis. When the eyelids are very swollen and the whites are very bloodshot; the eyelids may also appear red, and the eyes usually burn, sting, feel quite sore, and produce watery hot tears. Symptoms are worse with heat and better when the eyes are bathed in cold water.
- Mercurius vivus. For discharge that is puslike and irritating; when the person is restless at night and has night sweats.

You may also use Euphrasia (Eyebright) as a homeopathic eyewash: fill an eyecup with sterile water and add two drops of the tincture; use to wash the eye(s) three to four times a day. Or use Eyebright tea.

Dosage

Choose the remedy from the above list that most closely matches your symptoms. Administer following the Rule of Three (page 55). If the remedy does not prove to be effective, repeat the same process with the next homeopathic remedy that most closely corresponds with your symptoms.

Important Precautions

If you are presently taking allopathic drugs, or are under medical treatment for a specific medical condition, it is essential to consult your homeopath or allopathic doctor before administering homeopathic remedies. Medical care should also be sought if the conjunctivitis lasts more than a couple of days, especially if the patient is an infant; if the redness is concentrated around the pupil, or pupils are of unequal size; if the eyes are very painful or sensitive to bright light; if the vision is affected; if the eye has been injured or there is a foreign object in it that you are unable to remove, or if the discharge increases and gets thick, yellow, and looks like pus.

CONSTIPATION

Constipation—difficult, incomplete, or infrequent bowel movements—is one of the many side effects of too much "civilization." Contributing factors are a diet that overemphasizes processed foods such as white flour and sugar, cheese, and meat, plus too little exercise, and too much tension and stress. Sometimes travel, with its multitude of changes, also brings temporary constipation until we adjust.

You may be surprised (and relieved) to know that being "regular" doesn't mean having a bowel movement every day. "Normal" bowel movements may occur three times a day, or every three days—or anything in between. "Irregularity" is anything that is not regular for *you*. Even if the stools temporarily change in size, color, consistency, or frequency, it's usually no cause for concern. You may feel sluggish and bloated, but minor temporary irregularity is not harmful to your health and should respond to and be prevented by the General Homeopathic Home Care measures listed below. If you are very uncomfortable try the homeopathic medicines as well.

However, a prolonged and noticeable change in bowel habits may be a sign of serious disease, such as cancer or other intestinal illnesses. A tendency to chronic constipation means the bowels and nervous system are out of kilter and should be evaluated by a professional health-care practitioner.

General Homeopathic Home Care

The following guidelines will help prevent simple constipation in the future; they may also help you overcome a current case of sluggish bowels. Try to avoid taking strong laxatives, even occasionally; but if you must, use either psyllium seed (Metamucil is a well-known product), which is a bulk laxative, stewed prunes or prune juice, or an enema to get things moving again. But be aware it is all too easy to become dependent on these artificial means—which, like any crutch, weaken the system and prolong the problem.

- Eat plenty of fresh fruits, vegetables, and beans to add natural fiber to your diet. Fiber (roughage) is not absorbed in the intestine and acts as a sponge to hold water, creating a bulkier, softer stool, which stimulates bowel contractions and easier, more frequent passage.
- Drink lots of fluids, especially plain water, or fruit juice diluted with water, to work with the

fiber; sodas, coffee, and large quantities of black
or orange pekoe tea are not recommended.
- Adding pure bran (oat or wheat) to your diet is
not advised unless recommended by a nutrition
specialist. It's better to eat whole grains such as
oatmeal, Wheatena, and brown rice, which naturally contain bran.

Homeopathic Remedies

The following are the most commonly used homeopathic remedies for treating acute constipation:

- Calcarea carbonica. For someone who experiences no urge to move the bowels, and the stool
just sits in the rectum. For constipation following a large hard stool and then diarrhea that is
full of undigested food and smells sour; this
form of constipation may feel better to the person in contrast to the diarrhea. Calcarea helps
the body digest and assimilate food.
- Hepar sulphuricum. For constipation that follows another acute symptom such as a cold, a
cough, or an earache.
- Lycopodium. For stools that are difficult to pass
and are hard, or that feel as though much remains behind; when there is a lot of flatus.
- Natrum muriaticum. For small round stools that
are difficult to pass; when there is an unfinished
feeling after a bowel movement; when symptoms
are worse during the menstrual period. Natrum
helps the body correct any water imbalance.
- Nux vomica. For stools that are large and hard;
when the desire to pass stool is constant but not

successful; for an unfinished feeling with stools
that are small; the constipation may alternate
with diarrhea; when constipation is related to a
lack of exercise or pregnancy.
- Sepia. When the person has a weak feeling in the
rectum; the stool is hard and large, the abdomen
feels full and bloated, and straining to pass stool
is unsuccessful; when the constipation is associated with pregnancy or menstrual periods.
- Silica. For people who have difficulty passing
stools, even with straining; when there is a burning pain after a bowel movement; when stools
are hard and large and may be partially expelled
and slip back in because the muscles in the
bowel are weak.

Dosage

Choose the remedy from the above list that most
closely matches your symptoms. Administer following
the Rule of Three (page 55). If the remedy does not
prove to be effective, repeat the same process with the
next homeopathic remedy that most closely corresponds with your symptoms.

Important Precautions

If you are presently taking allopathic drugs, or are under medical treatment for a specific medical condition,
it is essential to consult your homeopath or allopathic
doctor before administering homeopathic medicines.
Medical care should also be sought if you have not had
a bowel movement in twenty-four hours *and* you have
severe or unusual pain; if the constipation has lasted

more than two weeks; if your stools are consistently black, gray, or white; if your eyes or skin are yellowish (jaundiced); if you alternate constipation with diarrhea; if blood accompanies the stools; or if constipation is accompanied by very thin stools, abdominal pain, and bloating or unexplained weight loss.

COUGHS

Coughing is a reflex that acts as a defense mechanism. An irritation or obstruction in one of the breathing tubes triggers the mechanism, which creates a strong upward rush of air. This explosive movement forces the irritating or obstructing material out of the tube. Coughing also helps to aerate the lungs and reorganize the breathing mechanisms.

Coughing often accompanies viral or bacterial infections: these include colds, influenza, croup (harsh barking cough in young children), laryngitis, bronchitis, and pneumonia. Other causes are a postnasal drip often related to allergies—mucus from the nose drains into the breathing tubes, causing an irritating tickle. Smoking cigarettes causes continual irritation of the tubes and is the number-one cause of coughs. In addition, the bodymind doesn't necessarily distinguish between a physical and an emotional or social irritant resulting in a cough. Babies and young children tend to swallow small foreign objects or accidentally inhale bits of food and such, which may lodge in the chest and trigger the coughing reflex.

In contrast to allopathy, homeopathy does not try to suppress the coughing reflex, since it represents the body's best efforts to expel something harmful, whether viruses, bacteria, or irritants, from breathing passages. Rather, homeopathic medicines make coughing a more effective healing tool so you no longer need it and it disappears quickly on its own.

See also "Colds," "Fever," or "Sore Throats" if the cough accompanies one of these conditions.

General Homeopathic Home Care

- Home care is similar to that for colds; see that section for details, especially if the cough is due to a cold. It's helpful to rest, drink fluids, and try to cough up any phlegm; increasing the humidity in the room thins the mucus and makes it easier to expel—this is particularly essential treatment for children with the croup. Drinking hot beverages also liquifies mucus. Rest is even more important because a cough is a deeper illness than a cold.
- Herbal lozenges help relieve the tickling of dry coughs; some studies show zinc lozenges slowly dissolved in the mouth also speed the progress of a cough.

Homeopathic Remedies

There are many homeopathic remedies used to treat coughs. The most commonly used are:

- Allium cepa. For the early stages of a dry, painful cough stimulated by a tickling in the larynx; hoarseness may accompany the cough; the symptoms are worse in cold air and better in a warm room.

- Nux vomica. For coughs that are dry, tickling, or racking and come on in fits; the larynx may tickle or feel raw, and there may be soreness in the chest; the symptoms are worse in the cold and during the early morning hours or after getting up; they are better after a hot drink.
- Bryonia. A very common cough remedy for dry, racking coughs that come on in fits and disturb sleep. There is usually pain in the chest and abdomen from coughing; the cough is worse with any kind of movement, including breathing, eating, or drinking, although a sip of water may bring temporary relief; symptoms are better with fresh air or lying on the most painful side (usually the right side).
- Phosphorus. This is used for many types of coughs; the cough is usually dry at night, but may be loose and phlegmy during the day; there is usually chest pain or a feeling of a heavy weight on the chest; the larynx may feel raw; the cough is worse with movement, changes in temperature, and cold or fresh air; lying down, particularly on the left side, makes the cough worse, and the person may be awakened by the need to cough; symptoms are better with warmth.
- Spongia. This is often the remedy of choice for harsh coughs and the croup; the cough is dry, barking, and often compared with the sound of sawing through a dry log; the cough may wake the person at night; symptoms are worse during the day and with excitement, talking, or exercise; they are better with eating and drinking.
- Antimonium tartaricum. When there is rattling

of mucus, but little phlegm can be raised; especially useful in children.

There are many other medicines that homeopaths use to treat coughs; if none of the above symptom pictures match the cough, you may want to study the mini-materia medica and compare the following remedies' general characteristics: Pulsatilla, Aconite, Hepar sulphuricum, Arsenicum, Lachesis, Ipecac, and Rhus toxicodendron.

Dosage

Choose the remedy from the above list that most closely matches your symptoms. Administer following the Rule of Three (page 55). If the remedy does not prove to be effective, repeat the same process with the next homeopathic remedy that most closely corresponds with your symptoms.

Important Precautions

If you are presently taking allopathic drugs, or are under medical treatment for a specific medical condition, it is essential to consult your homeopath or allopathic doctor before administering homeopathic medicines. Medical care should also be sought if the cough began suddenly and violently in a child who does not have a cold and who may have swallowed a foreign object; if it occurs in an infant under three months of age; if rapid breathing, difficulty breathing, or wheezing accompanies the cough; if it is severe and doesn't respond to home care in two days; or if there is prolonged high fever or extreme weakness.

DIAPER RASH

As the name suggests, this skin condition arises from our society's custom of keeping our babies' bottoms covered with diapers at all times. As a result, the infant's tender skin becomes irritated from the urine and dampness trapped in the covering. Infrequently changed diapers and the use of plastic pants promote diaper rash.

Diaper rash may remain a simple irritation, or the weakened, inflamed skin may allow a fungus or bacterial infection to take hold. The Candida fungus is often involved: this type of rash starts as small red spots, some of which may appear beyond the diaper area as far away as the chest. The spots grow into patches and the patches spread toward each other. Bacterial infections cause telltale fluid-filled blisters.

Diaper rash usually takes several days to clear up completely; it should improve with the General Homeopathic Home Care measures and homeopathic remedies within two days.

General Homeopathic Home Care

The goal of home care is to keep the area clean, dry, and exposed to the air as much as possible.

- Change diapers frequently and stop using plastic pants.
- Leave diapers off as much as possible.
- Wash, rinse, and dry the affected area thoroughly, using gentle, unperfumed soap. Pat dry with a soft towel; as an extra measure, you may use a hair dryer set on warm to make sure all

moisture evaporates (test the heat level on yourself first).
- If you use cloth diapers, wash them in a mild
soap and rinse them well; soap or detergent residue may add to the irritation.
- Try various protective barriers such as Calendula ointment, cornstarch, or baby powder.

Homeopathic Remedies

Diaper rashes should respond to the General Homeopathic Home Care measures; but if your baby seems
very miserable and an infection may be involved, try
these commonly prescribed remedies:

- Belladonna. For skin that is red and inflamed
and feels hot, but does not ooze.
- Arsenicum. For diaper rashes that itch and burn
and symptoms that are relieved by a warm bath
or compresses. The skin is cracked, raw, and
oozes fluid.
- Hepar. When there seems to be a bacterial infection, marked by pimples or pus; especially useful
if there is a foul odor that smells like old cheese.
- Sulphur. For a rash that itches severely and is
aggravated by a warm bath; when there may be
a bacterial infection with pimples or pus.
- Chamomilla. For babies who are extremely irritable and inconsolable.

Dosage

Choose the remedy from the above list that most
closely matches the baby's symptoms. Administer fol-

lowing the Rule of Three (page 55). If the remedy does
not prove to be effective, repeat the same process with
the next homeopathic remedy that most closely corresponds with the symptoms.

Important Precautions

If your baby is presently taking allopathic drugs, or is
under medical treatment for a specific medical condition, it is essential to consult your homeopath or allopathic doctor before administering homeopathic
remedies. Medical care should also be sought if the
condition does not improve after forty-eight hours, despite home care and homeopathic remedies; if the rash
has spread beyond the diaper area; or if there are blisters.

DIARRHEA

Diarrhea is an effective way for the body to get rid of
harmful substances such as viruses, bacteria, and tox-
ins. The mechanism slows the absorption rate of fluids
in the bowels, causing the intestines to contract force-
fully and rapidly. As a result, the loose or watery stool
is expelled, along with the harmful or symbolic or emotional substance it contains.

Diarrhea is a common symptom of gastroenteritis
(inflammation of the stomach or intestinal lining), flu,
or ear infection. Spoiled or contaminated food and
medications may also cause the body to react this way.
Anxiety, especially fear or the excessive desire to please,
can stimulate diarrhea as a way to relieve the uncomfortable inner turmoil.

Diarrhea is usually accompanied by some cramping, gas pains, or abdominal discomfort. Transient or isolated incidents of loose bowel movements and associated symptoms are not cause for concern; they usually resolve themselves quickly. Frequent, prolonged diarrhea poses the danger of dehydration, especially in infants when it is accompanied by vomiting and sweating due to fever. General Homeopathic Home Care, perhaps combined with a homeopathic remedy, usually helps the digestive tract return to normal.

General Homeopathic Home Care

Home care revolves around replacing lost fluids and slow, gentle reintroduction of easily digested foods.

- Limit eating for up to twelve hours after the first symptoms of diarrhea appear. This avoids stimulating the digestive system, which could cause more diarrhea.
- Gradually introduce clear liquids to replace the water the body has lost. Water, diluted fruit juice, bouillon, rice water (use double the usual amount of water and drain after cooking), are examples. Special replacement liquids containing minerals are available in pharmacies for use with infants. Jell-O, pure fruit juice, and Popsicles may also be tolerated.
- Next, introduce bland solid foods that tend to slow down the bowels. Think "BRAT": Bananas, Rice, Applesauce, and Toast.
- Avoid fatty foods, hard-to-digest foods, and milk and milk products, although nonfat yogurt may be tolerated.

- Offer fluids often to young children who may only want small amounts.

Homeopathic Remedies

The homeopathic remedies most commonly prescribed for diarrhea are:

- Arsenicum. When the diarrhea is violent and the person has severe pain in the abdomen; when stools are smelly and watery and cause burning pain; when diarrhea causes exhaustion; the symptom is worse after eating or drinking, and during the night; when the cause is food poisoning. (See also Nux vomica for food poisoning or overindulgence.)
- Colocynthis. When diarrhea accompanies cramping pains relieved by warmth and pressure (the person may press his fist into the abdomen or double over); stools are liquid or jellylike or pasty; stools are frequent and small; when symptoms are worse after eating and may be caused by anger.
- Bryonia. Most often used for diarrhea that occurs during the summer after eating too much fruit; stools are mushy and symptoms are worse in the mornings and during movement.
- Veratrum album. For violent, copious, uncontrollable diarrhea with cramps that may be sharp or aching; violent vomiting often accompanies the diarrhea; hands and feet are icy cold, but the person perspires, and he may be very hungry.

- Mercurius vivus. For severe urging and nausea before passing stool; when there is urging after passing stool; the person feels chilly but has flashes of heat, and feels thirsty for cold drinks.
- Pulsatilla. For mild diarrhea resulting from starchy or rich, fatty foods, and sometimes fruit; stools are changeable in character, but may be green and covered with mucus. This diarrhea gets worse after eating, at night, and indoors, and improves with fresh air.

Dosage

Choose the remedy from the above list that most closely matches your symptoms. Administer following the Rule of Three (page 55). If the remedy does not prove to be effective, repeat the same process with the next homeopathic remedy that most closely corresponds with your symptoms.

Important Precautions

If the person is presently taking allopathic drugs, or is under medical treatment for a specific medical condition, it is essential to consult your homeopath or allopathic doctor before administering homeopathic remedies. Medical care should also be sought if the diarrhea continues for three days. Watch for signs of dehydration, especially in infants and young children; this requires professional evaluation and can occur in twelve to twenty-four hours in adults and eight to twelve hours in children. A professional should also be consulted if the stools are black or bloody; if there is severe abdominal pain; or if there is unusual vaginal bleeding or persistent pain in women of childbearing age.

EARACHES

Earaches can happen at any age, but most often occur in children. The average child experiences at least one ear infection by age six, and some children are plagued by a series of ear infections. In children and adults, ear infections come in two varieties:

- *Otitis media* is an infection of the middle ear, the space behind the eardrum. Colds and allergies often lay the groundwork for middle-ear infections by narrowing the eustachian tube that leads from the middle ear to the nasal passages. The ear fluids that normally drain through the tube into the throat accumulate in this space, causing blockage and a comfortable environment for bacteria to grow in. Young children are particularly vulnerable because their tubes are so small and short. In children, symptoms are ear pain, fever, crying and fussiness, pulling the ears, restless sleep, and temporary hearing loss. The eardrum may rupture and allow a discharge to flow out. The rupture usually heals completely in a few weeks with no permanent consequences. Homeopathic remedies provide a safe, effective way to avoid antibiotics, which can weaken defenses and encourage further ear infections.
- *Otitis externa* is a skin infection of the ear canal that leads from the outer ear in toward the ear-

drum. Also related to bacteria, this is a shallow infection and less serious than otitis media. "Swimmer's ear," common in summer and among year-round serious swimmers, is a form of otitis externa. Symptoms are redness, inflammation, itchiness, and pain when the outer ear is moved, such as occurs when the earlobe is tugged.

General Homeopathic Home Care

• Learn to evaluate and diagnose ear infections. Ask your health-care professional to show you how to use an *otoscope* (available at pharmacies) to examine the ears of family members.
• As with any infection, rest helps the healing process.
• Consuming plenty of fluids helps keep secretions fluid and replaces water lost through perspiration.
• Moist heat, as from a hot towel or washcloth, or a hot water bottle, may soothe pain. Some people find cold relieves pain.
• For outer ear infections, moisten a piece of cotton fluff in Hypericum tincture (10 drops diluted in $\frac{1}{2}$ cup of water), Burow's solution, or a half-vinegar/half-water solution. Insert the cotton gently into the ear canal and allow it to remain for two to six hours. Rinse with plain water. This helps rid the ear of scaling and accumulated pus.
• Avoid inserting objects to clean out stopped-up

or pus-filled ears. This only drives the material in farther and may puncture the eardrum.

• Flush out packed-in wax with a syringe filled with warm water or hydrogen peroxide diluted with four parts water.

Homeopathic Remedies

The following are the most commonly used homeopathic remedies used to help heal earaches of all kinds:

• Pulsatilla. For a child who may cry or weep with pain, but is weak rather than irritable and angry; for earaches that develop during a cold, especially if there is a loose cough and/or thick nasal discharge.

• Belladonna. When the earache comes on suddenly and brings intense pain in the ear, which may spread to the neck or face; this remedy is best used when pus has not yet formed. (Ferrum phosphoricum is appropriate for cases that are similar to those requiring Belladonna, but less intense.)

• Chamomilla. For a child who is very irritable, screams and cries, and doesn't like to be touched; there is rarely a discharge from the ear.

• Silica. When a cold precedes the earache. Children who need Silica are particularly weak and tired and prefer to be warm; their ear might itch, and they may have a discharge from their ear and nose.

• Hepar sulphuricum. The symptoms resemble

those for Silica, but the child is angry, feels
chilly, and is worse at night.
- Mercurius vivus. The symptoms also resemble
those of Silica, except the child feels worse with
warmth and at night; he may perspire profusely
and have bad breath.

Dosage

Choose the remedy from the above list that most
closely matches your child's symptoms. Administer following the Rule of Three (page 55). If the remedy does
not prove to be effective, repeat the same process with
the next homeopathic remedy that most closely corresponds with the symptoms.

Important Precautions

If your child is presently taking allopathic drugs, or is
under medical treatment for a specific medical condition, it is essential to consult your homeopath or allopathic doctor before administering homeopathic
remedies. Medical care should also be sought if homeopathic care and remedy fail to improve an earache
within twenty-four hours in a young child, or in two to
three days in an older child or adult. Get medical care if
there is extreme weakness, severe pain, or stiff neck; if
there is any swelling, redness, or pain behind the ear;
if there is fever accompanied by a profuse ear discharge; or if there is hearing loss that extends beyond
two weeks. Have the ear examined by your homeopath
or physician three weeks after successful homeopathic
treatment to make sure the healing is complete.

FEVER

Fever is usually a symptom that a viral or bacterial infection has taken hold; these include colds, flu, earaches, diarrhea, cystitis, and common childhood diseases such as chicken pox, mumps, and measles. Although fever may be the only sign, or the major symptom, of an illness (especially during the early stage), the height of a person's temperature does not necessarily indicate the seriousness of the disease.

Fever, like all symptoms, has long been considered by homeopathy to be a positive sign that the body is defending itself from infection. Conventional medicine is finally realizing that fever has many beneficial functions. It speeds the metabolism so more blood, oxygen, and nutrients are available and waste products are carried away more quickly. The extra heat slows down the invading organism and makes it more vulnerable to the germ-fighting components of the immune system. This powerful, natural defense mechanism is usually not a cause for concern and in most cases it should be left alone to do its job during an acute illness.

Homeopathic home care helps keep the person more comfortable and supports the healing efforts of the body. In certain circumstances, a well-chosen homeopathic remedy offers a safe, effective way to reduce a fever by helping it to be a more effective healing tool. Consider adding a homeopathic remedy if: the fever is very high for a prolonged period of time (over 102 degrees Fahrenheit for more than an hour), or reaches 104 degrees Fahrenheit; if a child has had a febrile seizure in the past; or if the person is becoming depleted from the fever or is very uncomfortable.

(Note: If a child has a febrile seizure, do not become

unduly alarmed. Seizures usually last only one to five minutes, and rarely last longer than twenty or thirty minutes or cause permanent harm. Seizures are the body's reaction to a fever, which in certain children causes the brain to send inappropriate signals to the muscles. The body may stiffen, the hands and feet may beat rhythmically, the eyes may roll back and the head jerk. If the child vomits during a seizure, turn the child on his or her side to avoid inhalation of the vomit.)

If the fever accompanies other distinct conditions and symptoms, refer to those sections as well, such as "Flu," "Coughs," or "Sore Throats."

General Homeopathic Home Care

- Learn how to take a person's temperature to confirm and evaluate the severity of a fever. Oral thermometers work best for most individuals; rectal thermometers or axillary (armpit) thermometers work best in young children.
- Resting and drinking plenty of fluids support the body's healing efforts and replace fluids lost through sweating.
- A poor appetite is to be expected, so do not force foods. Small, bland, easily digestible meals are best.
- Protect the person from drafts and make sure she doesn't become chilled.
- A sponge bath is a natural way to relieve a fever. Sponge the person with tepid water for about twenty minutes. The water evaporation will cool the skin and the blood flowing close to the surface, bringing the overall temperature down. Finish by patting dry, and make sure the person

is protected from drafts during the procedure so
he or she doesn't get chilled.
- Sometimes just sponging the face and neck, plus
perhaps one limb at a time, will increase the person's comfort considerably.

Homeopathic Remedies

The following remedies are commonly used to treat
fever:

- Aconite. When the fever has come on suddenly
after the person became chilled; if symptoms include restlessness and anxiety and are worse at
night; if the person feels hot on the inside but
chilly on the outside; kicking the covers off is a
common trait, as is unquenchable thirst.
- Belladonna. For the person who radiates heat
and whose face is red and flushed; he may be
delirious, excitable, and have hallucinations;
there may be no thirst. The symptoms are worse
in the afternoon, evening, and night. (Ferrum
phosphoricum is the remedy of choice when the
symptoms are similar to those indicating Belladonna, but are less intense.)
- Nux vomica. When the person feels very chilly
and wants to stay completely covered; when
symptoms are accompanied by backache, and
alternate with chills and shivering. Symptoms
are worse in fresh air and drafts, and with movement.
- Pulsatilla. People who need Pulsatilla alternately
burn with fever and feel cold with chills; they
want to be uncovered one moment and covered

up the next; they tend to be whiny, weepy, and changeable; symptoms are worse toward the end of the day and during the evening.

- Mercurius vivus. For creeping chilliness, when the person is uncomfortably chilled, restless, or sweaty, especially at night.

Dosage

Choose the remedy from the above list that most closely matches your symptoms. Administer following the Rule of Three (page 55). If the remedy does not prove to be effective, repeat the same process with the next homeopathic remedy that most closely corresponds with your symptoms.

Important Precautions

NEVER give aspirin to a child who has fever that may be due to chicken pox, as aspirin increases the risk of a serious liver and brain disease known as Reye's syndrome. If the person is presently taking allopathic drugs, or is under medical treatment for a specific medical condition, it is essential to consult your homeopath or allopathic doctor before administering homeopathic remedies. Medical care should also be sought if a baby under six months of age has a fever; an older baby has had a fever for more than twenty-four hours that hasn't responded to homeopathic home care or remedies; the fever is over 105 degrees Fahrenheit in a person of any age; a child has had a febrile seizure during a past or the current illness; there are signs of dehydration.

FLU

Flu, or influenza, is a viral infection that is sometimes confused with a cold. Both affect the upper-respiratory system, but the flu is generally caused by different types of viruses that make you feel sicker than the typical cold virus does. Colds and flu share some symptoms—runny or stuffy nose, sneezing, sore throat, and cough —but flu generally also inflicts a high fever, fatigue, and a weak, ache-all-over feeling.

Conventional medicine offers a wide array of antiflu drugs that override symptoms and trick us into thinking we feel better, but do not enhance real healing. Flu symptoms, though discomforting, should not be suppressed because they help the body expel the virus and encourage us to take it easy so we can devote our energy to getting better. As is the case with all viral infections, homeopathy offers real help in terms of strengthening the body's response to the current infection as well as future infections. During the devastating influenza epidemic of 1917–1918, homeopathic care was much more successful at saving lives than was conventional care.

Refer to other sections of this book, such as "Coughs," "Colds," "Earaches," and "Sore Throats," to see if there are other remedies that more closely correspond to the person's total symptom picture and general characteristics. Sometimes acute gastroenteritis—a bacterial or viral infection of the digestive system—is called a "stomach flu." If you suspect a stomach flu, see sections on "Diarrhea," "Abdominal Pain," "Fever," and "Food Poisoning."

General Homeopathic Home Care

Home care is similar to that for colds, coughs, and fever. These gentle, effective measures include getting adequate rest, drinking fluids to avoid dehydration, inhaling steam or water vapor, and eating small meals.

Homeopathic Remedies

There are many homeopathic remedies suitable for home treatment of flu. The most commonly used are:

- Gelsemium. For flu sufferers whose main symptoms are fatigue, extreme weakness, a heavy feeling in the limbs, and muscle pain; their eyeballs may ache and their eyelids feel heavy; they may feel chills along their back, and feel chilly generally. Symptoms are worse with exertion because of weakness, and the person has little thirst.

- Bryonia. People who benefit are irritable and achy and do not want to be moved or disturbed because of pain; they may have headaches that are worsened by almost anything: touch, movement, eating, talking, moving the eyes. Coughing is often a symptom, as is thirst for cold liquids; symptoms are worse in warm rooms and better in cool air.

- Rhus toxicodendron. For flu primarily characterized by extreme exhaustion and pains in the joints, bones, and legs; paradoxically, the person feels restless, and worse if he lies still for long; accompanying symptoms include sleeplessness, nervousness, chilliness, thirst, sweating, and dry, hoarse throat. Symptoms are worse with initial movement, but better with continued movement such as a walk in the fresh air.

- Combination remedies. There are two highly effective commercially available combination remedies available—Oscillococcinum and Flu-Solution—which can be taken two to three times a day for the first symptoms of flu. These often nip the flu in the bud when taken early on. They are not useful for established flu.

Dosage

Choose the remedy from the above list that most closely matches your symptoms. Administer following the Rule of Three (page 55). If the remedy does not prove to be effective, repeat the same process with the next homeopathic remedy that most closely corresponds with your symptoms.

Important Precautions

If you are presently taking allopathic drugs, or are under medical treatment for a specific medical condition, it is essential to consult your homeopath or allopathic doctor before administering homeopathic remedies. Medical care should also be sought if the flu drags on for two weeks despite home care and homeopathic remedies. Professional advice is needed if any of the symptoms become severe, especially if cough is severe or fever returns after going away.

FOOD POISONING

Food poisoning can result from a variety of things: eating spoiled food that contains harmful bacteria, shellfish contaminated with toxic chemicals or parasites, insecticide-sprayed fruits and vegetables, or poisonous plants and mushrooms. The infamous ptomaine poisoning is caused by a staphylococcal enterotoxia (a bacterium) growing in foods high in protein (meat, fish, poultry, eggs) that have been improperly stored or handled.

Food poisoning causes sudden unpleasant symptoms of nausea, vomiting, and diarrhea—sometimes all at the same time—which effectively purge the body of the offending substance. Attacks can be quite violent, intense, and unrelenting; but they also usually resolve themselves in three to twenty-four hours, leaving you exhausted but on the road to recovery. Homeopathy can help speed the recovery time—sometimes cutting it in half.

See also "Diarrhea," "Motion Sickness," and "Abdominal Pain."

General Homeopathic Home Care

There is little you can do during the active phase of acute food poisoning—the symptoms are so intense, involving, and short lived. Afterward, when your digestive system has calmed down, home care revolves around replacing lost fluids and slow, gentle reintroduction of easily digested foods.

- Limit eating for up to twelve hours after the first symptoms of food poisoning appear.

- Gradually introduce clear liquids to replace the water the body has lost. Water, diluted fruit juice, bouillon, rice water (use double the usual amount of water and drain after cooking), are examples. Special replacement liquids containing minerals are available in pharmacies for use with infants. Jell-O, pure fruit juice, and Popsicles may also be tolerated.
- Next, introduce bland solid foods. Think "BRAT": Bananas, Rice, Applesauce, and Toast.
- Avoid fatty foods, hard-to-digest foods, and milk and milk products, although nonfat yogurt may be tolerated.
- Offer fluids often to young children who may only want small amounts.

Homeopathic Remedies

The homeopathic remedies used specifically when the symptoms are due to food poisoning are:

- Arsenicum. Usually the homeopathic remedy of choice for food poisoning, especially when the suspected culprit is spoiled meat. The nausea, diarrhea, and vomiting is intense, and the person can barely stand the thought, sight, or smell of food. In addition, the person wants small sips of water, and the illness often begins between 11:00 P.M. and 2:00 A.M.
- Nux vomica. This is the other classic remedy for food poisoning. In this case, the person feels as if there is a stone in the stomach, and vomits or wants to vomit but can't. There is often accom-

panying colic and diarrhea, and the symptoms
often start after 4:00 A.M.
• Lycopodium. When the food poisoning is due to
shellfish, particularly oysters.

Dosage

Choose the remedy from the above list that most
closely matches your symptoms. Administer following
the Rule of Three (page 55), administering the first dose
during a pause in the vomiting. If a dose is expelled
during vomiting, repeat the dose. If the remedy does
not prove to be effective, repeat the same process with
the next homeopathic remedy that most closely corresponds with your symptoms.

Important Precautions

Learn to recognize the signs of serious, life-threatening
oral poisoning, which occurs rarely with foods and
more often with medicines, insecticides, household
cleaners, and paint or paint solvents. Call your local
poison-control center if you suspect serious poisoning
has occurred. In addition, call a physician if symptoms
persist, and watch for signs of dehydration. If you are
presently taking allopathic drugs, or are under medical
treatment for a specific medical condition, it is essential
to consult your homeopath or allopathic doctor before
administering homeopathic remedies.

GERMAN MEASLES

German measles, or rubella, is a viral infection. It is usually mild and harmless in children, and lasts only a few days; thus it is sometimes referred to as the three-day measles. The symptoms include a short-lived low-grade fever, mild fatigue, a runny nose, swollen lymph nodes at the back of the neck, and a rash. The rash may assume a variety of forms, but usually begins on the face as tiny flat or slightly raised red spots. It then spreads to the torso and finally the limbs; meanwhile it is already fading from the face. In many cases, rubella doesn't cause a rash and mimics a simple cold or mild flu. Older children and adults who catch the German measles may experience joint pain that starts on the third day of the illness and lingers for some time afterward.

While rubella is no cause for concern in children and most adults, pregnant women who become infected in their first trimester may suffer greatly: their child stands a fifty-fifty chance of having birth defects. These include mental retardation, cataracts (cloudy lens of the eye), heart conditions, and a cleft palate.

General Homeopathic Home Care

There are no special steps to take for people with rubella, since it is such a mild infection. Bed rest is not required, although activities may be toned down for a day or two. Anyone with rubella, however, should be kept away from women who are pregnant—or who might be pregnant, since a pregnancy may not be evident during the first month or two.

Homeopathic Remedies

The following are most often used to treat German measles:

- Aconite. If symptoms come on suddenly; when there is fever, or restlessness, or the face is flushed. Aconite is usually given on the first day that symptoms appear.
- Belladonna. For times when the symptoms are similar to those for which Aconite is recommended, but the restlessness is replaced with dullness or delirium.
- Ferrum phosphoricum. When the symptoms appear more gradually; when fever and red spots appear on the cheeks but there is no general flushing; when the person feels chilly but sweats.
- Pulsatilla. When the illness includes nasal mucus or a loose cough. (Hepar sulphuris is more appropriate if the cough is harsher and croupy.)

Dosage

Choose the remedy from the above list that most closely matches your symptoms. Administer following the Rule of Three (page 55). If the remedy does not prove to be effective, repeat the same process with the next homeopathic remedy that most closely corresponds with your symptoms.

Important Precautions

If you are presently taking allopathic drugs, or are under medical treatment for a specific medical condition, it is essential to consult your homeopath or allopathic doctor before administering homeopathic remedies. Medical care should also be sought if the condition persists for more than seven days; if other severe symptoms of deepening illness occur, such as earache, or cough with chest pain; or if spiking fever or an increase in weakness occur as the days go by.

GRIEF AND SADNESS

Grief and sadness are part of everyone's life, because at some point we all lose someone or something we care about. It could be the death of a loved one or a pet; the loss of a job and thus our income and identity; the end of a relationship and thus the loss of a spouse, lover, or friend; we may be the victim of a violent crime such as a rape or mugging; we may need to move away from our home and experience the grief called homesickness.

Homeopathy has several remedies that support our own healing efforts during times of such acute crises. These remedies are able to soothe us when our feelings are still new, and thus at their most raw and painful. The expression of these natural feelings helps heal the injury of the loss and releases us to face the future with better balance.

General Homeopathic Home Care

We all have different ways and different timetables for recovering from important losses. Some of us bounce back right away; others need more time to heal. There is no "right" way, but the following suggestions have helped many people weather the emotional storm:

- As with all symptoms, suppressing grief and sadness is not healthy in the long run. Generally, it is better to acknowledge your loss and talk to another person or persons in a safe, supportive environment.

- Remember: emotions help you heal, so don't "beat yourself up" for feeling the way you do. Take the time to pray, meditate, contemplate, and honor your loss.

- The more important and deeper the feeling of grief, the more likely that unhealed losses in the past are being stirred up. But even this can be helpful because it brings up issues that are still bothering you and should be dealt with in order to restore balance.

- Listen to your own individual needs: Do you feel better when you are left alone, or are in the company of others? Might you find comfort in talking to people who share similar experiences and feelings? If so, seek out a support group or peer counselor who understands what you are going through. Often short-term counseling is all a person needs to get through a difficult period.

Homeopathic Remedies

The most often used homeopathic remedies for grief and sadness are:

- Ignatia. This is the most common remedy for the first stages of grief; for the person who weeps, sighs loudly, and doesn't sleep well because of her anguish. Especially helpful for sudden grief, and for use during and after hospital visits and funerals.

- Pulsatilla. For the person who weeps openly and freely, is helped by sympathy and comfort, is irresolute and dependent, desires change, and weeps while talking about her feelings.
- Natrum muriaticum. For the person who weeps in private, or for those who are sad but cannot weep and bravely dry their eyes and suppress the healing tears of sorrow.
- Nux vomica. For the person who complains, moans, and groans; for those who are sad and irritable, or taciturn and grumpy as if adverse to everything. The person may drink too much alcohol and give herself a hangover; she feels better if she has something to do.
- Cocculus. For the sad and weepy person who is sensitive and easily offended; she dreads every new piece of news and doesn't like to be contradicted.

Dosage

Choose the remedy from the above list that most closely matches your symptoms. Administer following the Rule of Three (page 55). If the remedy does not prove to be effective, repeat the same process with the next homeopathic remedy that most closely corresponds with your symptoms.

Important Precautions

If you are presently taking allopathic drugs, or are under medical treatment for a specific medical condition, it is essential to consult your homeopath or allopathic doctor before administering homeopathic remedies. Medical care should also be sought if crisis symptoms last for more than a week; if the suffering person talks about suicide; or if she uses alcohol or drugs and wants to drive a car while intoxicated.

HEADACHES

Almost everyone has had a headache at one time or another: this symptom is the most common complaint heard in doctors' offices and in day-to-day life. Some people are more prone to headaches than others, an indication that the symptom represents an individual's way of reacting to some form of stress.

When headaches are frequent and painful they may be a sign of serious disease and require professional evaluation. Homeopathy considers pain to be more than an alert mechanism that helps us identify times and places of distress in our body. Pain helps us modify our behavior to soothe the uncomfortable sensation in the short run. In addition, pain directly stimulates a healing effort to overcome the source of the disturbance. In homeopathy, every pain is welcomed because it is a sign of disharmony and encourages us to grow and change.

In most cases homeopathic home care and remedies have much to offer the person who suffers from the occasional mild headache, whether the cause is tension, something in the diet, or exposure to a toxic substance. There are two main categories of headaches: muscle contraction or tension headache; and vascular or migraine headache.

Muscle Contraction (Tension) Headache. This is the most common type of headache and usually feels like a dull ache with some tightness and tenderness at the temples, around the forehead, or where the skull meets the neck. The tension may be due to mental stress from, for example, overwork, or the mundane stress of everyday life, such as being stuck in congested traffic. A tension headache may also be the result of physical stress, such as too little sleep, a long, tedious drive, or poor posture. Sometimes both mental and physical stress are involved, as when sitting at a desk or straining at a computer for long periods of time in order to meet a deadline. Under stress conditions, the body reacts by tightening the muscles in the scalp, jaw, neck, shoulders, and back; eventually the muscles protest from the constant contraction; they become sore and the blood vessels that feed them constrict. In some cases, a temporomandibular joint problem (TMJ) may be the culprit; this misalignment of the jaw joint just in front of the ears requires a professional evaluation.

Vascular (Migraine) Headache. Migraine is a French word derived from the Latin word *hemicrania,* which means "pain in half of the head." This type of headache does usually affect only one side of the head, bringing severe throbbing pain. Migraines consist of two phases. In phase one, the blood vessels constrict and the brain receives less blood, leading to an early-warning sign called an "aura." Most often the aura consists of visual disturbances such as visions of lights, bright or geometric shapes and lines, and "tunnel" vision. Other auras include sensations of a strange taste or odor, tingling, dizziness, slurred speech, ringing in the ears, and weakness in a part of the body. This phase may also include nausea, vomiting, chills, extreme fatigue. As the next phase occurs, the blood vessels open abnormally wide, which stimulates the nerves in the blood vessel walls. The pain begins, and is usually accompanied by extreme fatigue.

A migraine may last for hours or days, and most often affects women. Such headaches tend to run in families. Migraine may be triggered by hypersensitivity or allergic reactions to foods, alcohol, bright lights, loud noises, hormonal fluctuations such as occur with the menstrual cycle, and some drugs. Some vascular headaches are known as "cluster" headaches. Also called histamine headaches, they are related to the release of histamine in the body during an allergic reaction. The eyes tear and water, the nose runs, and one side of the head feels severe pain.

Other headaches. Many other factors can trigger symptoms of headache, including an infection such as cold or flu, or inflammation of a general illness such as arthritis. Headaches may also be part of the multiple symptoms of many chronic illnesses such as emphysema, colitis, anemia, and alcohol and drug abuse. Sinus problems (page 232) also cause headaches.

General Homeopathic Home Care

For Tension Headache

- Try to determine and relieve the source of stress that is causing the headache. Examples are: poor posture at work, noise, holding the telephone between the ear and shoulder, eyestrain or ill-fitting eyeglasses, and various emotional and social conflicts. Take frequent breaks, periodically look into the distance if you do close work, and get proper work equipment.

- Rest if the headache makes you tired, or is severe.
- Massaging the scalp, face, neck, shoulders, and back may help relieve a headache; regularly scheduled massages or body work may help prevent one. Wet, hot compresses or a hot bath reduces the muscle spasms and relaxes you all over.
- Experiment with relaxation techniques to help reduce and manage stress (see page 104 in "Anxiety and Fear.")
- Look for foods and beverages that may be associated with your headaches. Some people are sensitive to certain foods or combinations; some people get headaches when they skip a meal, or do not drink enough fluids. Many people have headaches as a withdrawal symptom when they suddenly cut out all coffee—it's better to taper off gradually.

For Migraine Headache

Migraine headache can be so severe that home-care measures (and most allopathic drugs) don't offer much help. Homeopathic remedies prescribed by a professional are the best source of relief and prevention. However, you may want to try the following:

- Biofeedback teaches you how to warm your hands by increasing the blood flow to them. This appears to be effective in relieving migraine headaches for some people.
- Try to discover what triggers your migraine—

several foods have been implicated, including chocolate, nuts, coffee, cheese, citrus fruits, and alcohol. Or think about stressful situations that you could avoid.

Homeopathic Remedies

For mild and moderate headaches the most commonly used homeopathic remedies are:

- Belladonna. For burning, throbbing, violent headaches that start suddenly; when the symptoms are worse from light, noise, any motion (but especially from bending down), cold or heat, during the menstrual period, or exposure to sun; when symptoms are better with lying down in a darkened room, pressure, or wrapping the head in a warm covering, or sitting down.
- Nux vomica. For a "splitting headache" brought on by too much food, alcohol, coffee, or mental strain, or too little sleep. Cold wind, damp weather, or the common cold are other causes that indicate Nux as a remedy. This is the typical hangover headache and may be accompanied by nausea, vomiting, and a funny taste in the mouth. The Nux headache is worse in the morning, after eating, and upon shaking the head; it is better at night, with excitement, and after getting up.
- Bryonia. For dull, steady, or heavy headaches that last all day and are located mostly behind the eyeballs (particularly the left one) and in the forehead; when the person is irritable; when

symptoms are worse with coughing, after getting up, and with even slight motion of the head or eyes; and when the headache is better with pressure and cold compresses.

- Pulsatilla. For "nervous" throbbing headaches that may affect just the forehead, or be one sided; they may be caused by overeating (and be accompanied by nausea or vomiting), be related to the menstrual period, or come about as the result of nervousness or excitement. The headache is worse in a hot, stuffy room; after eating, bending or lying down, blowing the nose, or vigorous activity such as running. It is better with walking in the fresh air and with pressure.

- Gelsemium. For heavy, aching, sore pain that begins in the back of the head and may spread to the forehead, or is felt over the right eye or temple. There may be visual disturbances or other accompanying symptoms common in migraine; the head feels as though a tight band were encircling it and the eyes feel heavy lidded. The symptoms are worse with motion, light, and noise, and better after napping or urinating.

- Ignatia. For congestive headaches after feeling anger or grief; the pain is worse from the odor of tobacco smoke, and may appear in small spots, like a nail being driven into the head.

Dosage

Choose the remedy from the above list that most closely matches your symptoms. Administer following the Rule of Three (page 55). If the remedy does not prove to be effective, repeat the same process with the

next homeopathic remedy that most closely corresponds with your symptoms.

Important Precautions

If you are presently taking allopathic drugs, or are under medical treatment for a specific medical condition, it is essential to consult your homeopath or allopathic doctor before administering homeopathic remedies. Medical care should also be sought when a headache is unusually severe; lasts more than three days; occurs frequently; is steadily worsening; is accompanied by a stiff neck or fever; or occurs after a head injury or after taking a medicine (including birth control pills). Also see a doctor if you have a headache that for the first time is accompanied by migraine symptoms.

HEMORRHOIDS

Hemorrhoids, also called "piles," are veins in the lower anus or rectum that have become enlarged and inflamed. As a result, there often is pain, tenderness, burning, and itching; you may also notice bright red blood on the toilet paper, in the toilet bowl, or on the stools themselves. External hemorrhoids (outside the anal opening) appear as soft purplish lumps; internal hemorrhoids are not visible.

Factors that increase the likelihood of hemorrhoids include overeating, which causes pressure in the abdominal veins; prolonged constant sitting, which encourages the blood to pool in this area; and straining during a bowel movement, which usually accompanies hard, compacted stools. Anything that increases the pressure in the abdomen—such as straining at lifting weights, tension and anxiety, and pregnancy and labor —can encourage hemorrhoidal symptoms.

Hemorrhoids generally disappear within a week or a few days. They may leave a small scar or flap of tissue called a "tag." Homeopathic home care and remedies can treat and help prevent this annoying but harmless condition without resorting to the surgical removal or "rubber band" constriction technique favored by allopathy.

General Homeopathic Home Care

- Keep the anal area clean to minimize irritation and itching. Witch hazel–soaked "wipes" sold in drugstores are a handy, gentle way to cleanse away fecal debris.
- Sitz baths, in which you sit or squat in a few inches of warm water, soothe and cleanse the area thoroughly.
- To prevent hemorrhoids, avoid overeating and avoid straining to have a bowel movement, which puts pressure on the blood vessels in the anal area. Avoid coffee and highly seasoned foods, which can irritate the tissues. Avoid and treat constipation (see "Constipation"). If you have a sedentary job, take frequent breaks to walk around, and be sure to get enough exercise —both of these help maintain good blood circulation.

Homeopathic Remedies

Avoid allopathic hemorrhoid preparations that contain a local anesthetic (read the label and look for an ingredient ending in *-caine*); this can relieve pain temporarily but slow healing. The most commonly used homeopathic remedies are:

- Witch hazel is an herbal used specifically for shrinking inflamed hemorrhoids and rebuilding the strength and tone of the veins. In addition to using as a cleanser after passing stool, you may also use it as a wet dressing. Soak a washcloth or paper towel with witch hazel diluted in an equal part of water and apply to the hemorrhoid; allow to remain in contact with the inflamed area for ten to fifteen minutes. Repeat two to three times a day. There are also homeopathic ointments that contain witch hazel. (Hamamelis is the botanical name for this homeopathic remedy.)
- Nux vomica. When hemorrhoids are mild to moderate; there may be no bleeding at all, and symptoms are worse in the morning, with cold air, and in tight clothing; itching tends to be relieved by applying cool water. Nux is best for people who are sedentary and depend on coffee, laxatives, or other drugs.
- Arnica. For hemorrhoids that occur following childbirth; when the symptoms are worse from touch, motion, or rest, and better from lying down.
- Belladonna. For hemorrhoids that are severely

inflamed, red, swollen, and painful; when there
is a lot of bleeding.

- Sulphur. When the hemorrhoids cause pain
  when walking, sitting, or passing stool; there is
  oozing moisture at the anus and itching morning
  or night.
- Pulsatilla. When the hemorrhoids are accompanied by stools that change in color or consistency; when there is oozing of fluid and itching;
  when the person is pregnant or going through
  puberty, and is weepy, thirstless, clingy, and sensitive.

Dosage

Choose the remedy from the above list that most
closely matches your symptoms. Administer following
the Rule of Three (page 55). If the remedy does not
prove to be effective after two or three days, repeat the
same process with the next homeopathic remedy that
most closely corresponds with your symptoms.

Important Precautions

If you are presently taking allopathic drugs, or are under medical treatment for a specific medical condition,
it is essential to consult your homeopath or allopathic
doctor before administering homeopathic remedies.
Medical care should also be sought if this is the first
time you have symptoms of rectal bleeding; if you notice a change in the usual pattern of hemorrhoid symptoms; if you have profuse rectal bleeding or bleeding
and symptoms that do not improve after one week; if
you notice lumps or swelling near the anus; if you de-

velop general symptoms of weakness, fever, or muscle aches. A professional should also be consulted if a child awakens with rectal pain—this is a sign of pinworms, which live in the rectum.

HEPATITIS

The liver is our main metabolic factory. All of the nutrients absorbed in our digestive tract go directly to the liver for processing, distribution, and storage. Hepatitis is an inflammation of the liver, and is characterized by yellowing of the skin and eyes (jaundice), extreme fatigue, and an enlarged liver that feels heavy or tender. Loss of appetite, queasy stomach, light-colored stools, and dark urine can occur as a result of the sluggish and incomplete work that is all the inflamed liver is capable of.

Hepatitis is a serious illness and requires medical diagnosis and evaluation. It has several causes, including most often a viral infection, which is passed in the stool via food or water (hepatitis A); or through blood or sexual contact (hepatitis B). Other causes are mononucleosis; alcohol poisoning; drugs; worms or other parasites; or blood transfusion of the wrong blood type. Hepatitis A has a slow onset, often with cold- or flulike symptoms and slow progression of symptoms; it usually occurs in young adults, who recover completely. Hepatitis B can appear suddenly and progress rapidly; or it may be low grade, chronic, and result in the death of liver cells, cirrhosis (scarring of the liver), and death.

Hepatitis requires a professional diagnosis and evaluation. Allopathy does not have any effective medicines to treat hepatitis; however, homeopathic remedies have been able to enhance recovery in may cases. Usually treatment is done by a professional homeopath; if you are unable to be treated by a professional homeopath, you may want to use homeopathic home-care and remedies, along with conventional medical care prescribed by a doctor.

General Homeopathic Home Care

- Rest is the best course of action for anyone with hepatitis.
- Eat well, regardless of your lack of appetite: choose low-fat foods and moderate amounts of protein to avoid taxing the liver.
- Keep coffee, spices, and allopathic drugs to a minimum. Avoid alcohol completely.

Homeopathic Remedies

The most commonly used homeopathic remedies are:

- Aconite. Best in the early stages of hepatitis if there is high fever, restlessness, fearfulness, and when the person moans with discomfort.
- Belladonna. Another early-stage remedy when there is fever; when there is intermittent liver pain; when symptoms are worse with breathing, sudden movement, and lying down on the right side.
- Bryonia. For sharp pains in the liver that are worse from any motion, and better when lying on the right side. The person has a bitter taste in the mouth and is thirsty. He suffers from full-

ness and bloating of the abdomen that feels like a weight in the stomach.

- Lycopodium. When the liver is sore and the pain extends to the back, and when the abdomen also feels sensitive to pressure; accompanying symptoms are a sense of fullness after eating a small amount of food, gas, bloating, and a rumbling stomach.
- Nux vomica. Nux is usually used in people with hepatitis who use large quantities of alcohol or drugs.
- Sulphur. When there is a weightlike pressure in the stomach, and the area is sensitive to pressure. The person is thirsty, hungry, has morning diarrhea and stools that smell like sulphur, and feels weak at 11:00 AM.
- Chamomilla. For hepatitis characterized by a dull aching pain in the liver that is not made worse by pressure, motion, or breathing. The person who benefits from Chamomilla is sensitive, irritable, and thirsty, and feels hot.
- Mercurius vivus. When the symptoms include the mouth, and the tongue is puffy and the gums are swollen and bleed easily. In addition to the liver feeling swollen, tender, and uncomfortable when the person lies on the right side, the stools may be light colored.

Dosage

Choose the remedy from the above list that most closely matches your symptoms. Administer following the Rule of Three (page 55). If the remedy does not prove to be effective, repeat the same process with the

next homeopathic remedy that most closely corresponds with your symptoms.

Important Precautions

If you are presently taking allopathic drugs, or are under medical treatment for a specific medical condition, it is essential to consult your homeopath or allopathic doctor before administering homeopathic remedies. Medical care should always be sought if you have signs of hepatitis (jaundice, dark urine, light-colored stools); or if you may have been exposed to hepatitis.

HERPES SIMPLEX

A herpes simplex infection is caused by susceptibility to the herpes simplex virus, which invades the skin and nervous system. Herpes simplex virus overgrowth causes blisters to form; Type 1 is usually involved in cold sores (see page 129 for this type of infection). Type 2 usually produces blisters in the genital area.

The blisters are tiny and appear in groups, which may merge into bigger blisters. They appear several days after a person has been exposed to the virus, and are itchy, painful, and can be extremely uncomfortable. Some people also suffer from fever and enlarged lymph nodes during the attack. Within one week after symptoms begin, the blisters crust over and start to heal.

Genital herpes is not in itself serious. Infections in teenagers may be associated with an increased risk of cervical cancer when they become adults, if the susceptibility and recurrent irritation of infection is not overcome. Herpes is generally thought to be spread by sexual contact and is highly contagious before and during an eruption. Once the virus has gained entry and has caused the initial eruption it can live on in the nerve cells. A person may be permanently infected and experience repeated attacks, which can be triggered by other illnesses, stress, or traumatic injury. But usually the attacks become less bothersome over time.

General Homeopathic Home Care

- Rest is recommended during an attack. Reducing stress levels may also help speed recovery, and may decrease the frequency and intensity of future eruptions.
- Keep the blisters clean and dry and wash gently with mild soap and water.
- Some people report that a five- to ten-minute hot tub bath speeds healing.
- Take 2 to 3 grams (2,000 to 3,000 milligrams) of vitamin C daily, in divided doses.

Homeopathic Remedies

Allopathic medicine has no cure for herpes. The drug acyclovir (used in ointment form or taken orally) may reduce the healing time of an initial attack. But it is less effective during subsequent episodes, has many side effects, and homeopaths believe it may drive the illness deeper and weaken the person, whose body doesn't have to learn to cope with the virus. Homeopathic remedies include Calendula or Hypericum tincture: dilute 10 drops in ½ cup water and apply several times a day to blisters that have opened. The most commonly used oral remedies are:

- Rhus toxicodendron. For genital herpes sores that burn and itch intensely; when there are also symptoms of general achiness that improve with movement, and the pain shoots down into the legs.
- Arsenicum. For genital sores that burn severely and feel better with applications of warmth. The person feels chilly, has a fever, and is thirsty for small sips.
- Mercurius vivus. For herpes sores that itch, exude pus, form a crust, and are accompanied by swelling of the lymph nodes in the groin. The person is restless, hot, and chilly, and has a fever and night sweats.
- Sepia. For itchy herpes with pain that stretches up into the vagina. If the person has Sepia symptoms but the eruption occurs during the menstrual period, Mercurius is the better choice.
- Urtica urens. This remedy (Stinging Nettle) may be made as a tea and used as a wet dressing; or drink two to three cups of the tea daily if you are not taking another homeopathic remedy.

Dosage

Choose the remedy from the above list that most closely matches your symptoms. Administer following the Rule of Three (page 55). If the remedy does not prove to be effective, repeat the same process with the next homeopathic remedy that most closely corresponds with your symptoms.

Important Precautions

Sexual contact should be avoided during a herpes attack, and during the *prodrome*—a tingling or itching sensation that many people feel a day or two before the actual blisters erupt—because the virus is most contagious at these times. Condoms offer some protection, but it is not guaranteed or complete. Herpes simplex 2 infections can be serious in newborns and infants or anyone who has a compromised immune system such as the elderly, the ill (including the person with AIDS), or people having cancer therapy. Great care must be taken to prevent their exposure to the virus. A person with an active infection should cover the blisters and wash his or her hands thoroughly before touching someone who is particularly vulnerable.

If you are presently taking allopathic drugs, or are under medical treatment for a specific medical condition, it is essential to consult your homeopath or allopathic doctor before administering homeopathic remedies. Medical care should also be sought if this is your first attack and you are unsure if it is herpes; if the attack lasts more than two weeks; if it becomes infected with bacteria; if you have repeated attacks that are not clearly less severe over time; or if you think you may have herpes for the first time and are in the third trimester of your pregnancy.

HERPES ZOSTER (SHINGLES)

As is the case with all types of herpes viruses, the herpes virus that causes chicken pox (varicella-zoster virus) lives on in the body in the nervous system. In most people who have had chicken pox, the virus remains dormant and never causes any problems. In some individuals, however, the virus is reactivated and the result is a skin rash called "shingles."

The rash comes about when the virus travels along the route of the infected nerve, multiplies, and forms telltale red blistery bumps. It tends to cover a large area and be extremely sensitive and painful. Typically, only one side of the body is affected, usually the torso or the face. The pain of a herpes zoster attack may precede the rash and persist long after the rash has subsided, which takes about a couple of weeks. Shingles may be triggered by anything that decreases overall vitality or weakens the immune system, such as prolonged illness, cancer chemotherapy or radiation therapy, severe malnutrition (such as occurs with anorexia), AIDS, or old age.

In most cases, a herpes zoster attack leaves no permanent effects, except perhaps for some scarring where blisters were severe; however, attacks may recur periodically when the trigger is present.

General Homeopathic Home Care

- Rest is important during the early stages of a herpes zoster attack, especially when it is accompanied by fever or other whole-body symptoms.
- Since blisters are easily irritated by clothing or bed linens, use nonstick bandages or special frames that help prevent direct contact with such fabrics.
- In some cases, pressure on the rash, such as from an Ace bandage, eases pain.

- Applying cool compresses also brings relief to some people.
- Take 2 to 3 grams (2,000 to 3,000 milligrams) of vitamin C daily, in divided doses.

Homeopathic Remedies

Allopathic medicine involves pain medicine, antihistamines, and other drugs in certain cases. Homeopathic remedies help heal inflamed nerve endings and reduce pain during the attack. The most commonly used remedies are:

- Rhus toxicodendron. When the attack affects a fairly small area and the rash is very itchy; the person feels worse with bed rest, and better with warmth and movement.
- Apis mellifica. For rashes that sting and burn painfully and are accompanied by swelling; the symptoms are worse from warmth and better from cold applications. Apis is indicated when the person is not thirsty and is restless.
- Arsenicum. When the attack causes intense burning pain and symptoms include restlessness, anxiety, and weakness out of proportion to the illness; the pain is worse at night, and from cold air; the person feels better with warmth.
- Lachesis. For a rash that is very dark colored and painful; the rash that responds to Lachesis often occurs on the left side of the body.
- Mercurius vivus. When herpes consists of moist vesicles that bleed easily and burn when they are touched; they may be infected, and form pus and

crusts. The person feels hot and has chills and
night sweats.

- Urtica urens. When the blisters are large and accompanied by swelling. This remedy (Stinging
Nettle) may also be made as a tea and used as a
wet dressing; or drink two to three cups of the
tea daily if you are not taking another homeopathic remedy.

Dosage

Choose the remedy from the above list that most
closely matches your symptoms. Administer following
the Rule of Three (page 55). If the remedy does not
prove to be effective, repeat the same process with the
next homeopathic remedy that most closely corresponds with your symptoms.

Important Precautions

If you are presently taking allopathic drugs, or are under medical treatment for a specific medical condition,
it is essential to consult your homeopath or allopathic
doctor before administering homeopathic remedies.
Medical care should also be sought for initial diagnosis
and evaluation of the cause of the outbreak; if the rash
is on the face, or near the eye; if it doesn't improve after
seven days; if there are signs of bacterial infection such
as pus; if there is severe pain.

IMPETIGO

Impetigo is a bacterial skin infection that usually is confined to the face and affects children more often than adults. It may begin around the nostrils or lips or on the cheeks and then spread locally. The sores are small and red at first, then form blisters that itch, break, ooze yellow liquid, and finally form honey-colored or darker crusts. Impetigo is easily spread to other people—especially from child to child and from there to entire families. Most people recover from this strep/staph infection, but sometimes complications, such as a kidney disease or a deepening skin infection, can occur.

General Homeopathic Home Care

- Prevent the spread of impetigo by avoiding children or adults who have the infection.
- Try to keep children from touching sores and instruct them to wash their hands if they do happen to touch them; adults should follow these instructions as well.
- Wash the sores with mild soap and water. Do not scrub vigorously to remove the crusts; rather, soak them with warm water to soften them.
- The infected person should use his or her own individual towels, wash cloths, et cetera, and, if possible, sleep alone.

Homeopathic Remedies

Allopathic medicines such as local or oral antibiotics drive the disease deeper. They kill the bacteria, removing the need for our body to take care of itself. Each time our immune system successfully heals an infection, it "remembers" how to do this and will be better able to heal the next infection. Antibiotics prevent our immune system from learning to control the bacteria, leaving us with the original weakness. Homeopathy, however, helps the body learn to fight the infection. Commonly used homeopathic remedies include:

- Rhus toxicodendron. For impetigo infections that are unusually itchy and consist of clusters of tiny blisters; symptoms are better when the person is moving and after a warm bath.
- Mercurius vivus. For sores that seem to penetrate deeply into the skin and bleed slightly as well as produce pus that smells; there may be swollen glands and the person feels hot and has chills and night sweats.
- Hepar sulphuricum. For sores that are painful when touched; there may be additional symptoms of swollen glands and irritability; the sores feel worse when exposed to cold.
- Arsenicum. When the sores burn with pain. Sores that best respond to Arsenicum tend to look dark and may ooze water or pus; the sores feel better when warmth is applied.
- Antimonium crudum. Best used when the sores merge to form larger areas and thick yellow crusts, and when they seem to worsen and spread after bathing; additional symptoms are irritability and a white-coated tongue.
- Calendula tincture. Dilute 10 drops in ½ cup of sterile water, apply with cotton ball, and allow to dry.

Dosage

Choose the remedy from the above list that most closely matches your symptoms. Administer following the Rule of Three (page 55). If the remedy does not prove to be effective, repeat the same process with the next homeopathic remedy that most closely corresponds with your symptoms.

Important Precautions

If you are presently taking allopathic drugs, or are under medical treatment for a specific medical condition, it is essential to consult your homeopath or allopathic doctor before administering homeopathic remedies. Medical care should also be sought if the sores are very large, painful, or numerous; if the person has fever, or feels ill or achy; if the infection is moving toward the eye; or if the infection has not improved after two to three days; or to initially diagnose the condition in a child.

INSOMNIA

Almost everyone has trouble falling or staying asleep once in a while, or wakes up tired in spite of having spent "enough" hours in bed. All too many of us—an estimated fifteen to twenty million Americans—experience chronic insomnia.

Occasional insomnia is usually due to temporary overexcitement or worry about a specific thing. The body is ready and willing to rest, but the mind is revved up and thoughts and feelings go round and round. Another common scenario is "poor sleep hygiene"—all those little habits and circumstances that interrupt normal sleep cycles, such as irregular bedtime and waking time, too much noise or light in the bedroom, drinking coffee or eating a big meal late at night. Also, a disease or condition may keep you awake or disturb your sleep because of physical pain or discomfort.

Insomnia can become a chronic and vicious cycle. The less sleep you get, the less well you are able to deal with stress, and the more difficult it is to fall or stay asleep. Chronic insomnia also may result from chronic anxiety, fear, tension, depression and other psychological problems, drug abuse and dependence (including sleeping pills), or other chronic illness that causes nighttime symptoms of pain and distress.

In natural medicine systems such as homeopathy, sleep is one of the important components a person needs to heal properly, and to restore and maintain physical and mental health. New studies show that chronic sleep deprivation, which may be due to insomnia, affects the immune system and our ability to stay alert and concentrate. Inadequate sleep may be responsible for poor productivity, irritability, and a large portion of accidents on the road, on the job, and at work. We are only now discovering how important healthy sleep is and how widely requirements vary from individual to individual. Some people can thrive on four or five hours (not to be confused with those who "get by" on a few hours but require five, six, or more cups of coffee to get going and keep going). Others need nine or twelve hours to feel and do their best.

If you are questioning the adequacy of your sleep, ask yourself: do you need an alarm clock to wake up every morning? If so, you are not getting adequate sleep. Do you wake up refreshed and energetic? If you are, then you needn't worry about getting enough sleep. Your "insomnia" means you are trying to fall asleep too early, or get up later than your body needs you to. However, if you do suffer from occasional acute insomnia, or sleep fitfully and wake up tired, homeopathic home-care measures and remedies can help you restore a normal sleep schedule and awaken refreshed rather than exhausted. Chronic insomnia due to physical illness or emotional imbalance requires professional evaluation and counseling.

General Homeopathic Home Care

- Avoid drinking alcoholic beverages in the evening—although they may help you fall asleep initially, a few drinks before bedtime will actually awaken you in the middle of the night.
- Avoid caffeine (in coffee, black tea, sodas, chocolate, and some allopathic drugs) for several hours before bedtime. Some people are so sensitive to caffeine that even an afternoon cup of coffee keeps them up at night. Smoking also disturbs sleep.
- Establish a regular bedtime and waking time and don't deviate even on the weekend or during vacations.
- Create a bedtime ritual that cues your body for sleep and disengages the mind from daytime problems and thoughts. Relax by reading, taking a hot bath, or listening to music. Some people relax with friends; others find even lively conversation too stimulating. Watching TV may

be relaxing, but can also be stimulating, especially for children.

- Keep the bedroom for two things—sleep and sex. Using the bedroom for working overtime or paying bills signals the mind for activity, not relaxation. Some people find sex to be a pleasurable way to relax for sleep (although it could become habit forming!).

- Eat a light supper; you may find a snack such as toast or a small bowl of cereal relaxing. Some studies show eating a high-protein meal late in the day is detrimental to sleep, while carbohydrates encourage drowsiness.

- Establish a regular exercise routine, but avoid exercise at night, because it is stimulating.

- Some people find writing down the thoughts that are keeping them awake allows them to put the thoughts out of their minds long enough to fall asleep.

- Try using a relaxation technique (see page 106), which you can use both during the day and at night before retiring. Soothing relaxation tapes and soft music can be used as lullabies for grown-ups.

- Wear earplugs if your bedroom is noisy. Use a sleep mask and cover windows with heavy blinds or drapes if too much light comes through. Make sure the room temperature is comfortable and that there is adequate air circulation.

- Some people find daytime naps help; others find they make it more difficult to sleep at night, so experiment to see to which group you belong.

Homeopathic Remedies

Instead of "knocking you out" as habit-forming allopathic medicines tend to do, homeopathic remedies encourage the body to drift into a natural restful sleep.
The most commonly used remedies are:

- Nux vomica. For sleeplessness resulting from
  too much coffee, alcohol, or any other drug;
  from overexertion of the mind; from excess
  studying or working; the person is sleepy and
  falls asleep in the evening, but sleeps fitfully and
  awakens around 2:00 or 3:00 A.M. and is unable
  to fall asleep again for several hours.
- Pulsatilla. For someone who can't fall asleep until after midnight, and wakes up a few hours
  later; often a specific thought or memory keeps
  her awake and she may weep over sleep difficul-
  ties; the problem is worse in a warm room, and
  improves in the open air; the person may prefer to sleep with her arms thrown up over her
  head.
- Ignatia. This is most useful when the inability to
  sleep is caused by grief and the person sighs or
  yawns frequently; there may be the sense that
  sleep will never be possible, and the person
  whimpers while sleeping, and wakes up from
  muscle-jerking.
- Arsenicum. When the cause of sleeplessness is
  fear or anxiety; for people who are restless after
  midnight and cannot remain in bed, and who
  are chilly and want extra covers.
- Coffea. For insomnia due to sudden acute over-
  activity and overexcitement of body or mind,

following either a good event or bad event; also useful for people who stay awake because of drinking coffee. Coffea is a good illustration of "Like cures like"—small doses help cure what large doses cause.

- There are commercially available combination remedies that work well. Herbal drops of Passiflora (Passionflower) with or without Valerian can also be used as an occasional nontoxic sleep aid.

Dosage

Choose the remedy from the above list that most closely matches your symptoms. Administer following the Rule of Three (page 55). If the remedy does not prove to be effective, repeat the same process with the next homeopathic remedy that most closely corresponds with your symptoms.

Important Precautions

If you are presently taking allopathic drugs, or are under medical treatment for a specific medical condition, it is essential to consult your homeopath or allopathic doctor before administering homeopathic remedies. Medical care should also be sought if you experience insomnia for more than seven consecutive days; or if you have a painful medical condition that is keeping you from getting a good night's rest.

IRRITABILITY AND ANGER

Anger is an emotion that we often confuse with hatred or violence. Aggression and anger are part of our natural birthright as mammals, whereas hatred and the tendency toward violence are social, learned expressions based on fear, anger, and malice. Up to a certain point it is healthy to feel and express our anger. However, it does have its consequences, whether you are the one who is angry, or the one against whom the anger is directed.

Homeopathy can help you get through the ill effects of anger—for example, after experiencing a screaming match with your boss, your spouse, your parent, your teenager, or your friend. Such angry encounters can leave us shaking with indignation, sleepless, and obsessive about the conversation for days afterward ("I should have said . . ."). You may feel angry at yourself for having yelled back, or perhaps remorse over things you said. These are normal reactions and part of the healing process. Such acute reactions will subside gradually; they are not to be confused with those of the chronically angry person who is abusive and volatile in social situations and who requires professional help.

General Homeopathic Home Care

- Try to vent your anger through humor. Also, writing about your feelings in a journal is particularly helpful during a crisis.
- Recognize that it is healthy to vent your anger, but it is also healthy to say you're sorry.

Homeopathic Remedies

The most useful self-care remedies for anger and irritability are:

- Chamomilla. For anyone who is in a very emotional state, and has been for some time, and is now highly sensitive and irritable, mentally or physically. The person may rage violently, be difficult to please, and first wants this, and then that.
- Nux vomica. People who benefit from Nux vomica tend to be quarrelsome, irritable, aggressive individuals who hate to be contradicted and become angry when they are forced to reply to something they don't want to; their anger tends to be violent and they feel terrible if they hold it in.
- Hepar sulphuricum. When the slightest thing causes irritation and oversensitivity; when anger turns to violence. The person is touchy, chilly, and craves spices and strong-tasting foods. Although they share similar characteristics, the person who benefits from Hepar is not as impatient or fastidious over details as the person who needs Nux.
- Lycopodium. When the person is angry because he was contradicted, and is essentially low in self-confidence; Lycopodium is useful in children who are irritable and willful and prone to temper tantrums.
- Natrum muriaticum. For people who tend to suppress their emotions, especially anger and hurt, but then finally explode; they do not cry

easily, especially in public; the symptoms of irritability are worse just before menstruation; and the person is averse to consolation and may feel haunted by unpleasant events of the past.

- Sepia. For people who become angry and irritable when they are contradicted. This remedy is especially useful for women who may be irritable because they are worn out and exhausted from having too much to do. As with Natrum muriaticum, the person who benefits from Sepia is made worse by attempts at consolation.

Dosage

Choose the remedy from the above list that most closely matches your symptoms. Administer following the Rule of Three (page 55). If the remedy does not prove to be effective, repeat the same process with the next homeopathic remedy that most closely corresponds with your symptoms.

Important Precautions

If you are presently taking allopathic drugs, or are under medical treatment for a specific medical condition, it is essential to consult your homeopath or allopathic doctor before administering homeopathic remedies. Medical care should also be sought if violence occurs; if alcohol or drugs are being used to subdue the anger; or if accidents are occurring.

LARYNGITIS

Laryngitis is an inflammation of the mucous membrane lining the voice box (larynx), along with a swelling of the vocal cords, which causes hoarseness or loss of voice. This acute condition usually arises during an upper-respiratory infection such as a cold, or from overuse of the voice. If laryngitis accompanies other cold symptoms, such as a cough or sore throat, refer to those sections in the book for additional information about home care and homeopathic remedies.

Chronic laryngitis is usually due to smoking or to chronic overuse or incorrect use of the voice. It may also be a sign of serious disease. Therefore, chronic laryngitis requires either a halt to smoking, less vocalizing, a professional's evaluation and advice about the correct use of the vocal cords, or, lastly, medical treatment.

General Homeopathic Home Care

- To soothe the inflamed larynx and encourage healing, inhale steam from a vaporizer, humidifier, or bowl of heated water.
- Rest the voice as much as possible.
- Drinking liquids may help ease pain; some people prefer cold and some prefer warm beverages.

Homeopathic Remedies

The most commonly used remedies for laryngitis are:

- Phosphorus. For hoarseness caused by overusing the voice and that is accompanied by pain. The larynx tickles while speaking, and the cough is worse while talking and in the cold air.

- Spongia tosta. For hoarseness accompanied by a dry, burning sore throat and a dry, barking cough. The larynx is sensitive to the touch and there is a feeling of having a plug in the larynx. Eating or drinking soothes the cough.

- Rhus toxicodendron. When the throat feels dry and tickles, and the loss of voice occurs from overstraining. There is hoarseness upon waking in the morning that improves with gentle use, and then worsens again at the end of the day.

- Hepar sulphuricum. When the loss of voice occurs after exposure to cold, dry wind. There is a dry, hoarse cough that appears when any part of the body is exposed to cold air or after eating something cold.

- Kali bichromicum. When the larynx tickles, and the mucus is sticky and gelatinous and difficult to bring up. The hoarseness is worse in the evening.

- Sulphur. When the throat feels raw and dry and there is a choking sensation; the voice is most hoarse in the morning upon awakening. The person flushes with heat, feels weak in the late morning, and is worse after bathing.

Dosage

Choose the remedy from the above list that most closely matches your symptoms. Administer following the Rule of Three (page 55). If the remedy does not prove to be effective, repeat the same process with the

next homeopathic remedy that most closely corresponds with your symptoms.

Important Precautions

If you are presently taking allopathic drugs, or are under medical treatment for a specific medical condition, it is essential to consult your homeopath or allopathic doctor before administering homeopathic remedies. Medical care should also be sought if swallowing is very painful; there is excessive dribbling of saliva or breathing problems in a young child; the laryngitis lasts more than seven days.

MEASLES

Measles is a highly contagious viral disease that most often occurs in childhood. Early symptoms resemble those of the common cold: fever, cough, runny nose, irritated and watery eyes, and general discomfort. As the disease progresses, the child's eyes become sensitive to light and telltale small red or white spots appear in the mouth, on the inside of the cheeks. When the rash appears, it consists of irregularly shaped pink to brownish-pink patches on the face, ears, and neck. Within twenty-four to forty-eight hours the patches darken and spread to the body, arms, and legs. The fever soon drops and the rash flattens, turns light brown, and starts fading in three to five days.

Most children recuperate fully from the disease and suffer no lingering effects. However, measles can be quite severe and sometimes there are complications such as ear infections, pneumonia, or—rarely—encephalitis (brain infection). Homeopaths believe these are consequences of suppressing the symptoms by use of allopathic drugs, rather than of the disease itself, which should be allowed to run its course.

Vaccination against measles in the measles-mumps-rubella (MMR) combination is a standard recommendation for children. Homeopaths generally remain skeptical about the routine use of all of the "baby shots," but this issue should be discussed with a well-trained homeopath and your pediatrician.

See also the sections on "Fever," "Coughs," and "Sore Throats" if these symptoms are predominant or severe.

General Homeopathic Home Care

- Rest in bed usually helps the body cope with the infection.
- Since measles reduces appetite, avoid forcing food, but make light meals such as toast, soup, or rice available.
- To reduce risk of dehydration from the fever, be sure the child drinks plenty of liquids.
- Administer extra vitamin C in the form of supplements in divided doses as follows: 125 milligrams per day for toddlers, 250 milligrams per day for preschoolers, 1,000 milligrams per day for preteens, and 2,000 to 3,000 milligrams for teens and adults.
- Keep the light in the room dim by lowering the blinds or drapes.
- Application of cool compresses may soothe the rash.
- Take measures to prevent the spread of this

highly contagious disease; it is spread by droplets from the mouth and contact with items contaminated with nose and throat secretions.

Homeopathic Remedies

The most commonly used homeopathic remedies for
measles are:

- Aconite. The remedy of choice when measles
  comes on suddenly and there is fever, restlessness, a dry cough, and thirst; best used during
  the early stages of the infection.
- Belladonna. Another good choice for measles of
  sudden onset when symptoms include fever,
  cough, eye inflammation, and a headache that
  throbs; may be used early in the disease or after
  the rash appears. The child may twitch and be
  unable to sleep; and the symptoms are worse
  from noise, light, or jarring.
- Gelsemium. For measles symptoms that come on
  slowly, and that include fever and headache (especially in the back of the head); the child typically feels heavy and drowsy, can barely keep
  her eyes open, and is not thirsty.
- Euphrasia. When a child with measles suffers
  mostly from symptoms of eye inflammation such
  as burning, itching, watering, and sensitivity to
  light, and coldlike symptoms of a runny nose
  and cough; other than these symptoms the child
  doesn't feel very ill and usually runs only a mod-
  erately high fever.
- Bryonia. When the symptoms appear slowly and
  include a bad cough, fever, and headache; the

rash takes a long time to appear; the chest hurts and muscles ache so much, the child doesn't want to move; the fever makes the mouth feel dry and the child is very thirsty for cold drinks.

- Pulsatilla. For the child who has a cough and other symptoms of the common cold; when she is weepy and irritable, and may be nauseated and have diarrhea. Pulsatilla is useful in the later stages of the infection, particularly when symptoms linger.
- Kali bichromicum. When symptoms are similar to those for Pulsatilla, but are worse and include thick, sticky discharges.

Dosage

Choose the remedy from the above list that most closely matches your child's symptoms. Administer following the Rule of Three (page 55). If the remedy does not prove to be effective, repeat the same process with the next homeopathic remedy that most closely corresponds with your child's symptoms.

Important Precautions

If your child is presently taking allopathic drugs, or is under medical treatment for a specific medical condition, it is essential to consult your homeopath or allopathic doctor before administering homeopathic remedies. Medical care should also be sought if the child has a severe headache, is extremely lethargic, is vomiting, or has a convulsion; is bleeding from the nose, rectum, or mouth or under the skin; has difficulty breathing; develops an earache; or if symptoms persist

beyond five days after the rash peaks. Measles in a child
under six months also requires professional care.

MENSTRUAL CRAMPS AND
PREMENSTRUAL SYNDROME (PMS)

Many women experience some form of discomfort before or during their menstrual period. Cramps, back
pain, bloating, swollen breasts, food cravings, acne,
mood swings, irritability, and fatigue are some of the
symptoms from which you may suffer each month.
Premenstrual syndrome (PMS) begins at or after ovula-
tion (usually around the middle of the menstrual cycle)
and may continue until the beginning of menstruation.
Many women continue to experience symptoms such as
cramps during menstruation.

While PMS has only recently been recognized by the
medical establishment as a valid health disorder (it used
to be that it was "all in our heads"), it's nice to know
that the syndrome has always been treated by homeopaths. Medical specialists now estimate that PMS affects more than 90 percent of fertile women at some
point in their lives. In some women the condition is so
severe that it disrupts work and social relationships.
Hormonal changes that happen throughout the menstrual cycle clearly influence PMS, but allopathic doctors differ in theories on the exact cause of PMS.

Allopathic medicines containing the chemical
ibuprofen reduce levels of prostaglandins, which cause
menstrual cramps. Some contain diuretics, which ad-
dress the bloating by artificially reducing excess water
in the tissues. But in homeopathy the entire system is

treated, not simply one or two chemical imbalances. PMS and severe menstrual cramping are related to hormonal function and reproduction and so are considered to be important and deep conditions by homeopaths. The crisis symptoms may be soothed by the self-care homeopathic measures and remedies listed below, but curative treatment usually requires a visit to an experienced homeopathic doctor.

General Homeopathic Home Care

- Take a warm bath or curl up with a hot water bottle. Drink hot herbal teas. Warmth increases your blood flow, and can relax your cramped pelvic muscles.
- Good nutrition helps. Cut out caffeine, alcohol, and salt from your diet. Caffeine can make you nervous, and worsen insomnia and pain. Alcohol and salt may contribute to menstrual bloating. Some women have also found that limiting dairy products can reduce their symptoms of PMS. Eating light and easily digestible meals (bland, low-fat cooked foods including vegetables, fruit, grains, fish, et cetera) throughout the day can also reduce that bloated feeling, as well as contribute to your overall health.
- Increase your intake of calcium and magnesium. Women taking calcium suffer less from cramps, and magnesium aids in your body's absorption of calcium.
- Exercise can help. Moderate activities such as walking and stretching alleviate menstrual cramps in many women.

Homeopathic Remedies

The most common homeopathic remedies indicated for women suffering from menstrual discomfort are:

- Belladonna. For acute cramps that may feel like bearing-down labor pains; for menstrual cramps in which bending over aggravates the pain; when pain is aggravated by motion of any kind.
- Pulsatilla. For PMS symptoms that include moodiness, sensitivity, depressions, and a tendency to cry; also relieves dizziness, nausea, diarrhea, headaches, and back pain; for many types of menstrual pain, especially if the woman moans or cries with the pain.
- Magnesia phosphorica. The best remedy for simple menstrual cramps that are relieved by warmth, pressure, or bending over, especially if the menses and pain are associated with lethargy.
- Colocynthis. For severe menstrual cramps that are relieved primarily by bending over, although warmth and pressure may also help; to relieve the irritability or anger during the period.
- Chamomilla. For symptoms based largely on your mood; soothes the anger and irritability that can accompany PMS and menses; also relieves cramps.

Dosage

Choose the remedy from the above list that most closely matches your symptoms. Administer following the Rule of Three (page 55). If after eight to twelve hours you are still experiencing pain, repeat the same process with the next homeopathic remedy that most closely corresponds with your symptoms.

Important Precautions

If you are presently taking allopathic drugs, or are under medical treatment for a specific medical condition, it is essential to consult your homeopath or allopathic doctor before administering homeopathic remedies. Medical care should also be sought if there is very severe pain or unusual pain in the pelvic area or abdomen, particularly if accompanied by fever or unusual vaginal bleeding (heavy, clotted, scanty, or none).

If severe menstrual cramps are not relieved by homeopathic remedies, don't give up on homeopathy. It still may work, so seek the advice of a professional who can treat this crisis episode of an underlying chronic illness. In addition, evaluation and diagnosis by a gynecology specialist is always useful in the treatment of severe, chronic menstrual disorders.

MONONUCLEOSIS

Mononucleosis is a viral infection that often mimics others such as strep throat or prolonged cold or flu. Symptoms are sore throat, inflamed tonsils, extreme fatigue, aches, and fever. The lymph nodes in the neck are swollen. For most people "mono" appears similar to a severe cold or tonsillitis, possibly with a cough and unusually severe weakness. For a few people, deeper illness develops, which includes an enlarged spleen and hepatitis (inflamed liver).

Although allopathic medicine doesn't have much to offer in the way of treatment, it is important to get a professional diagnosis. You need to know what you have so you can choose a specific homeopathic treatment to help your body learn how to recover and make sure the spleen and liver are not involved. Untreated, mononucleosis can result in long-term low-grade infection, weakness, illness, and months of debility.

General Homeopathic Home Care

- Rest as much as possible to allow your body to marshal its forces and focus on healing.
- Gargle with warm salt water to soothe your sore throat; to prepare, dissolve a pinch of salt in a six-ounce glass of pure water (chlorine free).
- Take 2 to 3 grams (2,000 to 3,000 milligrams) of vitamin C in divided doses throughout the day.

Homeopathic Remedies

Some of the remedies discussed under "Fever" and "Sore Throats"—especially Belladonna and Hepar sulphuris—are effective for mononucleosis. In addition, the following remedies are often used for this condition:

- Mercurius. Use this remedy when there is a sore throat, pus on the tonsils, tender, swollen glands, pain radiating into the ears, a foul mouth odor, a wet mouth, and drooling. Other typical symptoms that indicate Mercurius are profuse odorous sweating especially at night, creeping chilliness, thirst for cold drinks, and restless sleep—the person feels first too hot and then too cold, and wants the covers off and then back on.

- Lachesis. For mono with a sore throat, especially if it occurs on the left and the pain is worse from hot drinks. Lachesis is also indicated if the glands are swollen, and the pain in the throat and glands are worse from touch. The person can't bear to have his neck covered, or wear clothes that are tight at the waist. The liver is sensitive, there is a fever with hot flushes, and the person feels worse after sleeping.

- Kali bichromicum. When there is a sore throat, dry cough, with hawking of mucus that is especially difficult to expel in the morning. The person may feel weak and apathetic, have a low-grade fever and chills, and usually feels better from warmth.

- Cistus canadensis. This is the remedy for mono that is prolonged in spite of treatment with another remedy. The person has a sore, swollen, dry throat with pain that feels worse when he inhales cold air and better when he drinks liquids; he hawks mucus and has swollen glands; he has chills when exposed to the slightest bit of cold air.

Dosage

Choose the remedy from the above list that most closely matches your symptoms. Administer following the Rule of Three (page 55). If the remedy does not prove to be effective, repeat the same process with the

next homeopathic remedy that most closely corresponds with the symptoms.

Important Precautions

If you are presently taking allopathic drugs, or are under medical treatment for a specific medical condition, it is essential to consult your homeopath or allopathic doctor before administering homeopathic remedies. Medical care should also be sought if urine turns dark or jaundice develops, indicating hepatitis; the sore throat is severe and may require a strep culture; there is severe weakness or fever that lasts more than seven days. Do not engage in contact sports or vigorous athletics until a doctor has checked for an enlarged spleen, which is susceptible to rupture.

MOTION SICKNESS

In the car, boat, or airplane, some of us get dizzy, pale, and nauseous. We may break out in a cold sweat and lose our lunch, toss our cookies, or ditch our dinner. Collectively these queasy feelings are known as motion sickness, a condition that most scientists believe is related to imbalances in the inner ear. Visual stimuli and anxiety can contribute to the severity of the reaction.

General Homeopathic Home Care

- Stay away from unpleasant odors, such as engine fumes or strong food smells.
- Don't smoke. Smoking can contribute to nausea.

Nonsmokers should avoid being near people who are smoking.

- Eat in moderation. Stay away from foods that don't agree with you and avoid alcoholic drinks.
- Get some fresh air. Opening a car window may stave off a bout of nausea, as may taking short walking breaks.
- Start your trip out well rested. Being overtired can increase your risk of motion sickness.
- Position yourself defensively. In a car you are less likely to get sick in the front- than the back-seat. On a boat stay abovedeck and to the forward end, where there is less bouncing. And in a plane get a seat over the wing and avoid the tail, where there is more movement.

Homeopathic Remedies

Homeopathic remedies most frequently recommended for motion sickness are:

- Cocculus. The most common homeopathic remedy for nausea, vomiting, and dizziness; when symptoms are worse when you rise from a lying position, or from odor, noise, the thought of food, and being chilled.
- Nux vomica. The most readily available homeopathic remedy to treat motion sickness; for nausea, headache, and buzzing in the ears.
- Petroleum. For dizziness; for dizziness that precedes nausea and cold sweats; for nausea associated with pain in the stomach, head, or back; when increase in saliva accompanies nausea.
- Tabacum. For very severe nausea, cold sweats,

and violent vomiting; when symptoms are better in the open air and when the eyes are closed.

Dosage

Choose the remedy from the above list that most closely matches your symptoms. Cocculus is usually the most useful, but Nux vomica the most commonly accessible, homeopathic remedy for the treatment of motion sickness. Administer the remedy following the Rule of Three (page 55). If Cocculus does not prove to be the right homeopathic remedy for you, repeat the same process with the next homeopathic remedy that most closely corresponds with your symptoms.

Important Precautions

If the person is presently taking allopathic drugs, or is under medical treatment for a specific medical condition, it is essential to consult a homeopath or allopathic doctor before administering homeopathic remedies. As with any condition of vomiting, if the symptom is relentless and the person is unable to hold down fluids, he or she should be evaluated professionally for dehydration; this may occur after twelve to twenty-four hours in adults and eight to twelve hours in children.

MUMPS

This is an infection of the major salivary glands located just below and in front of the ears. Mumps mainly affects children and, less often, young adults. However, mumps may occur at any age. The symptoms are swelling at the jawline, which may appear on one or both sides. The swelling is usually painful, and is accompanied by fever, headache, and loss of appetite. Sometimes the ears ache as well. Symptoms are usually mild in children, but may be severe in adults. In many cases, someone may have mumps and not be aware of it because there may be no swelling at all.

Mumps is a viral infection that is carried in the saliva of the infected person and spread by airborne droplets or direct contact. This infection can be distinguished from swollen lymph glands (which are part of the circulatory and immune systems) because you will be unable to feel the edge of the jaw beneath the ear. In addition, chewing, swallowing, and eating sour foods such as pickles and lemons worsen the pain because they stimulate salivary glands.

General Homeopathic Home Care

- Since symptoms are usually so mild, bed rest is not generally necessary.
- Because mumps is contagious and can be serious in adults, keep the infected person away from adults who have never had mumps.
- Avoid spicy or sour foods, and foods that require a lot of chewing.

Homeopathic Remedies

The most commonly used homeopathic remedies for mumps are:

- Belladonna. For mumps that appear suddenly, this is the most often used remedy. There is fe-

ver, redness, and swelling, and there may be
sharp intermittent pains in the glands. The swelling may appear on the right side only.

- Pulsatilla. For the later stages of the disease, especially if the symptoms linger and the child is
weepy and thirstless; when she feels worse from
warmth and better in the open air.
- Mercurius vivus. For the child with offensive
sweat and breath, who has a bad taste in her
mouth, and who salivates profusely.
- Lachesis. When the parotid gland (below and in
front of the ear) is severely swollen, especially on
the left side, and is very sensitive to touch so the
person shrinks away when she is approached to
be touched. The person can hardly swallow, has
a sore throat, and the face is red and swollen.

Dosage

Choose the remedy from the above list that most
closely matches your symptoms. Administer following
the Rule of Three (page 55). If the remedy does not
prove to be effective, repeat the same process with the
next homeopathic remedy that most closely corresponds with your symptoms.

Important Precautions

If your child is presently taking allopathic drugs, or is
under medical treatment for a specific medical condition, it is essential to consult your homeopath or allopathic doctor before administering homeopathic
remedies. Medical care should also be sought if the

child has convulsions, extreme lethargy, or a stiff neck; if there is pain and swelling of the testicles in a male, or the breast or ovaries in a female; if there is pain in the abdomen, vomiting, dizziness, or difficulty hearing.

NAUSEA

(See "Abdominal Pain and Indigestion.")

NECK PAIN

(See "Back and Neck Problems.")

POISON OAK OR IVY

(See "Allergies: Contact Dermatitis.")

PROSTATITIS

As men grow older, they tend to have problems with the prostate, the walnut-sized gland that produces the fluid that carries sperm. The prostate lies close to the bladder, where urine is stored, and surrounds the urethra, the tube through which urine leaves the body.

Prostatitis is an inflammation and swelling of this gland. The symptoms of acute inflammation are an urge to urinate frequently, or a burning sensation during urination, difficulty starting to urinate, fever, weakness, and pain in the area of the prostate, which may spread to the genitals, pelvis, or farther up the back. It may feel as though there is a lump in the rectum. Acute prostatitis is due to susceptibility to a bacterial infection. Chronic inflammation sometimes occurs after an infection; symptoms are milder but return and linger. The chronic form of this condition may also develop when there is no bacterial infection.

Allopathic medicine treats prostatitis with antibiotics (in very acute cases, high-dose intravenous antibiotics are prescribed), but finds chronic prostatitis notoriously difficult to treat. Other medications may be used to relax the urethra, and antiinflammatory drugs to ease the pain. Homeopathy can help both acute and chronic prostatitis, but be sure to see a health professional before trying home care. The bacteria involved are sometimes particularly dangerous, and the symptoms may also indicate prostate cancer, a common disease in older men.

General Homeopathic Home Care

- Drink large amounts of fluids to dilute urine and help wash out the bacteria. Avoid coffee, black tea, and highly seasoned foods, which may cause further irritation.
- As with any acute infection, bed rest helps the body direct its forces toward healing.
- Men with chronic prostatitis can prevent the prostatic fluid from accumulating and worsening the inflammation by ejaculating every day or every other day. However, during an acute attack you should rest the prostate by avoiding ejaculation and sexual stimulation.
- "Kegel" exercises may also help in chronic in-

flammation. You can perform these yourself by contracting the muscles used to stop and start the flow of urine; hold each contraction for a few seconds and then relax. Do one hundred Kegels each day to encourage the prostate gland to empty its fluid. Alternatively, you may have the prostate massaged by a health professional.

Homeopathic Remedies

The most common homeopathic remedies for prostatitis are:

- Pulsatilla. When there are sharp pains around the prostate that radiate to the bladder and pelvis; there may be a discharge from the penis; the pain is worse after urination; the urethra burns during and after urination. Pulsatilla is most appropriate for men who are worried, sad, and need attention and comfort during the crisis of the illness.
- Lycopodium. When there is a sensation of pressure in the prostate; pressure is worse during and after urination; there may be sharp pains in the bladder and anus. The man has a constant urge to urinate, but he must wait for the flow to start and can't feel the urine as it passes.
- Kali bichromicum. For sharp, needlelike pain, burning after urination, and a thick, stringy discharge. The pain is worse from walking.
- Thuja. This is a great prostate tonic for men who have a constant urge to urinate; who start, then stop, and start again when urinating; or

who feel a sensation of trickling after urination. There may be pain after urination and prostate pain.

- Sepia. When there is a constant urge to urinate and the man has to wait for the urine to start; he feels anxiety and pressure in the bladder if he tries to hold in the urine; there may be a mucous discharge and pain in the urethra.

Dosage

Choose the remedy from the above list that most closely matches your symptoms. Administer following the Rule of Three (page 55). If the remedy does not prove to be effective, repeat the same process with the next homeopathic remedy that most closely corresponds with the symptoms.

Important Precautions

If you are presently taking allopathic drugs, or are under medical treatment for a specific medical condition, it is essential to consult your homeopath or allopathic doctor before administering homeopathic remedies. Medical care should also be sought if there is pain or swelling in the testicles, in the prostate or surrounding area; if you have had sexually transmitted disease; if you have trouble starting or maintaining urination, have a weak urine stream, or if you have a discharge from the urethra.

RINGWORM AND OTHER RELATED FUNGAL INFECTIONS

The skin can be susceptible to a variety of fungal infections. A fungus is a simple parasitic plant that depends on the skin for food. Ringworm (which is due to a fungus, not to worms) makes itself known as circular patches of rough, dry, slightly raised, slightly red skin. Athlete's foot, jock itch (the pubic region), and nail fungus infections may also occur; fungus may also attack the scalp, face, trunk, arms, and legs. Some infections look like small round spots that have lost their color and are most obvious in the summer because they do not tan. Other minor fungal infections appear as lightly scaled tan, pink, or white patches.

Fungus infections may or may not itch, and have varying degrees of contagion. They usually disappear by themselves eventually, but homeopathic home care measures and remedies can speed the process while avoiding powerful allopathic antifungal medicines. Nail infections develop slowly and can be healed, but usually an experienced homeopath is needed to help. If the fungal infection keeps coming back, or is persistent, you should have a general medical evaluation to help understand your individual susceptibility.

General Homeopathic Home Care

- The first rule of thumb is to remove the contributing factors: moisture and friction. Wash the affected area at least twice a day with mild soap and dry thoroughly. You may want to wash more often if the area becomes moist from perspiration, as for example the feet or genitals. A hair dryer set on low heat will help evaporate the last traces of moisture; hold the hair dryer at arm's length to avoid exposure to its electromagnetic field. Wear clean loose-fitting underwear and shoes (such as sandals) that allow air to circulate.

- Expose the skin to light as much as possible, since fungi love the dark.
- Decrease exposure to fungus by wearing shower shoes ("flip-flops") at health clubs, gyms, public pools, et cetera.
- Apply plain vinegar, diluted with an equal amount of water, to the infected area a few times a day, making sure the skin is dry before replacing your clothing.
- Use powder (corn starch or baby powder) in the folds and creases of your skin to keep it dry.

Homeopathic Remedies

Among the most commonly used homeopathic remedies for fungal infections are:

- Sepia. For ringworm that appears in isolated spots; the rash is dry, but the skin becomes rough and moist after scratching, and this somewhat relieves the itch. Sepia is a good remedy for the type of fungus infection that results in pale white, slightly scaly spots.
- Sulphur. For infections that are very itchy, and become more itchy from warmth, such as the warmth of a bath or a bed. The itch is worse and begins to burn after scratching.
- Arsenicum. For dry ringworm with rough scales;

the itch gets worse and the rash may become wet
after scratching. The person may pick at the
scale until it bleeds.

- Graphites. For infections that ooze thick amber
  fluid, especially after scratching, and the skin becomes thick and cracked. Graphites is indicated
  when the rash occurs in the folds of the skin.
- Tellurium. This is a hard-to-find remedy, but is
  useful for ringworm that is wet with tiny blisters, red, and itchy. The itch is worse at night in
  bed.

Dosage

Choose the remedy from the above list that most
closely matches your symptoms. Administer following
the Rule of Three (page 55). If the remedy does not
prove to be effective, repeat the same process with the
next homeopathic remedy that most closely corresponds with the symptoms.

Important Precautions

If you are presently taking allopathic drugs, or are under medical treatment for a specific medical condition,
it is essential to consult your homeopath or allopathic
doctor before administering homeopathic remedies.
Medical care should also be sought if the fungal infection doesn't begin to clear up in a week or two; if the
skin becomes red, hard, and tender, indicating a bacterial infection.

SCIATICA

(See "Back and Neck Problems.")

SEXUALLY TRANSMITTED DISEASES (STDs)

STDs are contagious diseases that spread through sexual intercourse or genital contact. They are becoming more and more common and include gonorrhea, syphilis, genital herpes (see "Herpes Simplex"), genital warts (see "Warts"), trichomoniasis (see "Vaginitis"), chlamydia, and acquired immunodeficiency syndrome (AIDS).

Many sexually transmitted diseases are serious. They cause painful symptoms, may lead to sterility, chronic scarring of the reproductive organs, and death. If you suspect you have a sexually transmitted disease because you have symptoms or because you have had unprotected sex with someone who may have a sexually transmitted disease, consult a health professional for diagnosis and treatment. Homeopathic treatment can be used along with allopathic treatment to speed recovery, or after allopathic treatment to strengthen the bodymind.

SINUS PROBLEMS (SINUSITIS)

Sinusitis is a swelling of the sinus cavities, the open spaces in our skulls above the eyes, within the nose, and inside the cheekbones. During a cold or allergic reaction (such as hay fever, a food reaction, or sensitivity to environmental irritants), the mucous membrane lining the sinus may become swollen. This blocks off the opening leading from the sinus to the nose, causing pressure, pain, congestion, headache, tenderness or a sense of heaviness behind the eyes and nose, and fever. Other conditions that may cause sinus problems are dental infection and a change in atmospheric pressure (as during air travel or a scuba dive).

Sinusitis may be mild or severe; acute; chronic; or recurring. When the sinuses become overwhelmed with a bacterial infection, symptoms worsen and there may be a pus-filled discharge from the nose. Sinusitis may affect only one side of the head, or both. Allopathic medicine treats sinus infections with decongestants, pain medication, antibiotics, and, in severe and recurrent cases, surgical drainage. Homeopathic measures and remedies can accelerate recuperation from sinusitis, without side effects of drugs or surgery. For additional information see also sections on "Colds," "Allergies: Hay Fever," and "Headaches."

General Homeopathic Home Care

- Take it easy and get rest, especially if the sinusitis is severe.
- Use a vaporizer, humidifier, or bowl of steaming water to loosen mucus and relieve sinus congestion. Wet, hot compresses applied to the painful area may also be soothing.
- Drink plenty of fluids to help liquify mucous secretions.
- As with all infections and allergies, take 2,000 to 3,000 milligrams (2 to 3 grams) of vitamin C every day, in divided doses.

Homeopathic Remedies

The most often used homeopathic remedies for sinusitis
are:

- Kali bichromicum. When sinus pain occurs primarily at the root of the nose, in the forehead
over one eye, and occasionally below the eyes.
There is a very thick puslike nasal discharge and
crusts. Symptoms may begin in the morning,
worsen by midday, and get better in the afternoon. The symptoms are worse from cold
weather, bending down, and any motion such as
walking; they are better from pressure, warmth,
and drinking warm liquids.
- Hepar sulphuricum. For pain that occurs primarily at the root of the nose; the entire head
may feel sore and bruised and sensitive to touch
or movement; symptoms are worse in cold air
and in the morning. There may be a thick, offensive nasal discharge.
- Silica. For sinus pain that is worse from the cold,
mental exertion, noise, motion, bending down,
or talking; it is better with pressure and warmth.
There is an irritating nasal mucus and crusts in
the nose.
- Phosphorus. For sinus pain in the cheeks, and a
pus-filled nasal discharge that may also contain
some blood.
- Nux vomica. When the nose feels inflamed,
there is a nasal discharge, and the nose stops up
at night.

Dosage

Choose the remedy from the above list that most closely matches your symptoms. Administer following the Rule of Three (page 55). If the remedy does not prove to be effective, repeat the same process with the next homeopathic remedy that most closely corresponds with the symptoms.

Important Precautions

If you are presently taking allopathic drugs, or are under medical treatment for a specific medical condition, it is essential to consult your homeopath or allopathic doctor before administering homeopathic remedies. Medical care should also be sought if the sinus pain is severe, or there is high fever or a smelly discharge; if there is an infection that doesn't improve with homeopathic care or remedies in forty-eight hours.

SORE THROATS

A sore throat can mean many things; most of them are not serious, and heal on their own. Sore throats may be noninfectious, or indicate an overgrowth of viruses or bacteria.

Noninfectious sore throats are usually related to a dry throat caused by breathing through the mouth, especially in winter when the air is heated and dry. Other conditions that lead to noninfectious sore throats include allergies and irritations; in these instances, excess mucus drips down the throat, causing irritation (postnasal drip). These sore throats subside once the conditions that caused them are out of the way.

Viral sore throats are often caused by the viruses that cause the common cold. These are rarely serious and respond to the same treatment suggested in the section on "Colds." Severe sore throats may be caused by the mononucleosis virus. This type mostly affects children and adolescents. It can be severe and often lasts quite a long time. (See the section on "Mononucleosis.")

Strep throat is short for streptococcus, the bacterium that causes many sore throats. Strep is likely to be the culprit only if there are no accompanying symptoms of a cold, such as runny nose, sneezing, stuffy ears, cough, and congestion. Another indication is that the throat pain is usually more severe and dominates the symptom picture, and the person feels sicker and has a higher fever. Strep is not necessarily serious, but it can lead to serious complications, so a professional diagnosis is usually recommended if you suspect strep. For example, rheumatic fever can cause permanent heart damage; kidney disease can also result from a strep infection. A less serious consequence of strep throat is scarlet fever.

Allopathic medicine has no treatment for viral sore throat. Bacterial infections such as strep throat may be treated with antibiotics. However, antibiotics will prevent rheumatic fever only if they eradicate all the bacteria and are begun within nine days of the onset of the disease; there is no proof that antibiotics prevent the strep-associated kidney disease. They do not affect symptoms or duration of a sore throat unless treatment begins within twenty-four hours of the onset. Antibiotics are therefore virtually useless for all sore throats, except perhaps in children or adults with a history of

rheumatic fever. These high-risk individuals are advised
to take them at the onset of any sore throat, without
waiting for the results of a throat culture to confirm the
diagnosis. If the person with a sore throat is a child in
school or an adult health worker, teacher, or child care
provider, it is important to do a throat culture to rule
out or confirm a contagious strep infection.

General Homeopathic Home Care

- Drink plenty of fluids to lubricate the throat.
- Increase the humidity of the air with a humidifier or vaporizer.
- Gargling with warm salt water (a pinch of salt
  dissolved in 6 ounces of chlorine-free water), or
  drinking hot lemonade sweetened with honey,
  may soothe a sore throat and flush away mucus,
  viruses, and bacteria.
- Zinc lozenges that are specifically designed to
  dissolve easily may help hasten recovery. Avoid
  eucalyptus or mentholated lozenges if you are
  taking a homeopathic remedy, since these could
  antidote the remedy.

Homeopathic Remedies

- Belladonna. Best used at the first sign of a sore
  throat, when symptoms appear suddenly and are
  accompanied by flushed skin and fever. Swallowing makes the throat feel worse, the throat
  feels dry, and the person does not want to drink
  liquids.
- Aconite. When symptoms appear suddenly, per-

haps after exposure to cold air or a draft; the throat feels dry and the person is thirsty; fever accompanies the sore throat, and the person may feel chilled.

- Mercurius. When the pain is severe, accompanied by fever, and the throat is red and swollen; the tonsils or throat may have white or yellow deposits of pus; there is increased saliva, pain radiating into the ears during swallowing, a mouth odor, fever with sweaty and restless nights. The person is easily chilled and overheated.

- Lycopodium. For sore throats that are worse on the right side; pain may spread from the right to the left; there is fever with chills. Throat pain is worse from cold air, but the person craves fresh air; the pain is better after a warm drink. Symptoms are generally worse in the late afternoon.

- Hepar sulphuris. This remedy is indicated when the throat pain feels like a splinter, with the sensation extending into the ears during swallowing. There is fever with chills from the slightest draft, and the person needs to hawk up mucus from the throat.

- Lachesis. For painful, swollen throats that are worse on the left side, or that spread from the left to the right. Symptoms are worse from drinking, particularly warm beverages, and worse in the morning or upon waking at night.

- Rhus toxicodendron. When the pain is severe and occurs after straining the throat by talking, singing, or exposure to cold, wet weather. The soreness may be worse in the morning and after initially swallowing, but improves with continued swallowing. The pain lessens with warmth and drinking warm beverages.

- Arsenicum. When the throat burns with pain and symptoms include chills, fever, thirst, fatigue, and restlessness. The sore throat feels worse from swallowing, cold beverages, and cold air; it feels better from warm beverages.
- Sulphur. Try sulphur when the symptoms linger or the first choice of remedy was not effective; when the throat burns, feels dry, and is better from drinking warm beverages. Sulphur is also indicated if the person is lethargic, and has bad breath and smelly sweat.

Dosage

Choose the remedy from the above list that most closely matches your symptoms. Administer following the Rule of Three (page 55). If the remedy does not prove to be effective, repeat the same process with the next homeopathic remedy that most closely corresponds with the symptoms.

Important Precautions

If you are presently taking allopathic drugs, or are under medical treatment for a specific medical condition, it is essential to consult your homeopath or allopathic doctor before administering homeopathic remedies. Medical care should also be sought if the pain is severe; swallowing is very difficult; there is a lot of saliva and drooling; there is difficulty breathing; the sore throat is accompanied by fever and doesn't improve in forty-eight hours with homeopathic treatment; or a strep culture is needed for public-health reasons to prevent a child from spreading a strep infection to other children in school or day care.

STYES

A stye is an infection of a sweat gland or oil gland of the eyelid, usually involving an overgrowth of staphylococcal bacteria. The infection forms a tiny red bump, which is tender. The stye develops a head in a few days, which opens and drains pus. Styes or similar bumps may form on the eyelid margins or under the lid and are rarely serious. Some styes may be related to rubbing the eye with a dirty hand, but recurrent infections are best treated with a constitutional homeopathic remedy that strengthens resistance to infection.

General Homeopathic Home Care

- Hot compresses, such as a clean washcloth soaked in hot water, encourage the stye to come to a head and pus to drain. Apply for ten to fifteen minutes every three hours.
- You may also use hot compresses of Calendula tincture, diluted 10 drops in ½ cup of water.

Homeopathic Remedies

The most often used homeopathic remedies for styes are:

- Pulsatilla. This is the most common remedy for this condition and usually hastens healing before pus has a chance to form.
- Hepar sulphuricum. For styes that form a lot of pus, and that are red and inflamed; the lid is sensitive to the touch and to cool air, and helped by application of heat. The pain may throb. Silica is used when the symptom picture is similar to that of Hepar—check the "Glossary of Homeopathic Remedies" for general symptoms.
- Sulphur. For people who form styes often; the lid burns, itches, and feels hot; the symptoms are worse with heat.

Dosage

Choose the remedy from the above list that most closely matches your symptoms. Administer following the Rule of Three (page 55). If the remedy does not prove to be effective, repeat the same process with the next homeopathic remedy that most closely corresponds with the symptoms.

Important Precautions

If you are presently taking allopathic drugs, or are under medical treatment for a specific medical condition, it is essential to consult your homeopath or allopathic doctor before administering homeopathic remedies. Medical care should also be sought if the vision is affected; there is fever, lethargy or headache; the stye does not improve within forty-eight hours of homeopathic treatment.

TEETHING

Some children produce their first teeth with little or no
noticeable discomfort. Others may be extremely uncomfortable: as their baby teeth erupt through the
gums, they experience pain, fever, colds, diarrhea,
moodiness, and sleeplessness. Their gums become sensitive, tender, swollen; they produce excess saliva; they
fuss and cry. As a result, the teething process can become a nightmare for the entire family. Homeopathy
can make a big difference in the teething experience, so
if home care doesn't help, see a professional homeopath
for treatment.

General Homeopathic Home Care

- A cold or frozen teething ring will give your
  baby something cold to gnaw on, and seems to
  relieve discomfort.
- Some babies prefer to chew on a clean moist
  cloth wrapped around chipped ice.

Homeopathic Remedies

The most commonly used remedies for teething babies
are:

- Chamomilla. This is the primary remedy for
  teething pain and sensitivity for babies who are
  irritable, restless, whining, thirsty, and hot. Typically, the child who benefits from Chamomilla
  wants things and then refuses them, and may
  angrily throw them across the room; she is not

easily comforted, but carrying and rocking her helps.
- Magnesia phosphorica. For teething pain in a child who complains; symptoms are better from warm drinks and warm compresses applied to the jaw.
- Calcaria carbonica and Silica. These remedies are often given for the tendency to delayed and painful teething; check the general characteristics described in the "Glossary of Homeopathic Remedies."

Dosage

Choose the remedy from the above list that most closely matches your child's symptoms. Administer following the Rule of Three (page 55). If the remedy does not prove to be effective, repeat the same process with the next homeopathic remedy that most closely corresponds with the symptoms.

Important Precautions

If your child is presently taking allopathic drugs, or is under medical treatment for a specific medical condition, it is essential to consult your homeopath or allopathic doctor before administering homeopathic remedies. Medical care should also be sought if your child is inconsolable, refuses to eat or drink, develops a fever, or appears to develop signs of an ear infection (see "Earaches").

THRUSH

Thrush is a Candida fungus infection of the mouth that is a common condition in babies and uncommon in adults unless their immune system is impaired. The fungus (or yeast) overgrowth looks like raised white patches on the tissues of the mouth. Along with other organisms, yeast organisms are present in the normal, healthy mouth, and usually only cause a problem when the individual is susceptible to infection.

General Homeopathic Home Care

- Eating plain yogurt with live yogurt cultures helps restore the balance of organisms in the throat and mouth.
- To prevent spread and reinfection clean and, if possible, sterilize toys that the child tends to put in her mouth.
- Avoid sugar and sweet drinks, which may encourage yeast overgrowth.

Homeopathic Remedies

The most useful homeopathic remedies for thrush are:

- Borax. For thrush infections that bleed easily; when the child produces excess saliva; or when she cries when nursing. Borax is also used for elderly people when thrush is caused by dentures.
- Mercurius vivus. When the child produces excess saliva, has bad breath, and perhaps mouth ulcers.

- Natrum muriaticum. When the tongue and gums have a white coating, the mouth feels dry, and the individual is thirsty.
- Sulphur. When the infection feels sore and burns; eating is painful.

Dosage

Choose the remedy from the above list that most closely matches your symptoms. Administer following the Rule of Three (page 55). If the remedy does not prove to be effective, repeat the same process with the next homeopathic remedy that most closely corresponds with the symptoms.

Important Precautions

If you are presently taking allopathic drugs, or are under medical treatment for a specific medical condition, it is essential to consult your homeopath or allopathic doctor before administering homeopathic remedies. Medical care should also be sought if the thrush recurs frequently; if the infection is severe; if thrush develops in any older child or any adult.

<u>URETHRITIS</u>

Urethritis is an inflammation of the urethra, the tube through which the urine passes from the bladder to the outside of the body; in men the urethra also carries semen. Because their urethra is longer, urethritis is more common and causes more severe symptoms in men than in women. In women, urethritis often accompanies vaginitis (see page 248) or cystitis (page 122), and prostatitis in men (see page 225).

Urethritis causes symptoms of burning, pain, and difficulty when urinating; frequent urination; and a discharge that may contain pus or mucus, which tends to be more noticeable in the morning. The condition is usually related to an overgrowth of sexually transmitted bacteria, most often chlamydia; in the male, urethritis is also a well-known sign of gonorrhea. Usually both sexual partners are infected, even if they both do not have symptoms. Sometimes urethritis is not a sign of infection, but rather of irritation, such as is caused by physical trauma or certain drugs such as marijuana; or it may occur after taking antibiotics for another infection.

Mild cases of urethritis respond well to homeopathy. (However, any new case of urethritis in men should be cultured to rule out a sexually transmitted disease.) If urethritis persists despite homeopathic self-care, it should be looked at by a physician, because it may spread to other people. If untreated, bacterial infections of the urethra can spread to other parts of the urinary tract and may cause sterility.

General Homeopathic Home Care

- Drink plenty of fluids to dilute the urine, stimulate frequent urination, and help rid the urethra of bacteria.
- Support your body's natural healing processes by getting enough rest, managing stress, and eating a healthy diet.

- Take 2 to 3 grams (2,000 to 3,000 milligrams) of vitamin C every day in divided doses.
- Avoid substances that might irritate the urethra further, such as coffee and spicy foods.

Homeopathic Remedies

The most commonly used homeopathic remedies for urethritis are:

- Apis and Cantharis. Either one of these remedies is useful for the first sign of inflammation accompanied by a discharge. Cantharis is best when there is severe burning and urgency before, during, and after urination; Apis is best if the pain is more like a stinging sensation.
- Pulsatilla. When the discharge is thick and yellow or green, and is nonirritating; when there is pain during urination and the flow starts and stops; when the person needs attention and comforting.
- Mercurius vivus. For discharges that are thick and puslike or mucuslike, and are accompanied by burning and inflammation (especially when beginning to urinate); for burning in the urethra when the person is not urinating; the symptoms are worse at night.
- Natrum muriaticum. For discharge that is clear and watery, or thick like mucus, or milky; or the discharge may look greenish, or dry to a yellowish color on the underwear. During or just after urination, there may be sharp or burning pain.

Dosage

Choose the remedy from the above list that most closely matches your symptoms. Administer following the Rule of Three (page 55). If the remedy does not prove to be effective, repeat the same process with the next homeopathic remedy that most closely corresponds with the symptoms.

Important Precautions

If you are presently taking allopathic drugs, or are under medical treatment for a specific medical condition, it is essential to consult your homeopath or allopathic doctor before administering homeopathic remedies. Medical care should also be sought if you suspect you might have a sexually transmitted disease, either because of specific symptoms, or because you have had sexual contact with someone who might have a sexually transmitted disease; if your symptoms are severe or have not improved in two days with homeopathic self-care.

VAGINITIS

A woman's vagina and cervix are anatomically designed to secrete fluids. These fluids vary according to the phase of the menstrual cycle, sexual excitement, and pregnancy. A discharge is not necessarily a sign of illness, but you should be aware of any changes in your normal vaginal secretions: the amount, the consistency, color, and odor, as well as any other symptoms such as inflammation and itching. Such changes are indications that you have vaginitis, an overgrowth of microorganisms.

Certain conditions can change the balance of normally present microorganisms in the vagina and encourage the overgrowth of one type over another. These include a weakened immune system (for example from stress or overwork), menopause, medications that cause a hormone imbalance, use of chemicals such as birth control products, and others. There are several types of vaginitis, caused by different organisms, and characterized by a variety of symptoms.

Yeast infections are probably the most common. Also called Candida or monilial infection, a yeast infection of the vagina is characterized by a thick whitish discharge that may look like cottage cheese and smells like baking bread. Yeast infections also can be maddeningly itchy and the external genital tissues become red and irritated. Yeast may grow out of control after a woman has been treated with a course of antibiotics for a bacterial infection, because the drugs also wipe out vaginal bacteria that kept the normally present yeast in check.

Bacterial infections may be due to a variety of different bacteria. This type of vaginitis is often referred to as nonspecific vaginitis and results in a white or yellow discharge; there may be symptoms similar to cystitis (see page 122), and lower back pain, cramps, and swollen glands in the groin. Chlamydia and gonorrhea are sexually transmitted bacterial infections that should be identified through a professional examination.

Trichomonas infections involve an amoebalike organism and are characterized by a thin, foamy yellowish or greenish discharge that smells offensive. Trichomonas is sexually transmitted and requires a professional examination to identify.

Noninfectious vaginitis may be due to irritation from chemicals (such as douches, diaphragm jelly, or spermicide), sexual activity, or a tampon that has been inadvertently left in. The vagina becomes red and swollen and may produce a discharge to rid the body of the irritation.

Vaginal infections, though annoying, are usually not dangerous. Homeopathic home care and homeopathic remedies can help strengthen the body and speed recovery. Some infections can be serious and result in infertility. If you have any doubts about the seriousness of your vaginitis, consult a health professional.

General Homeopathic Home Care

- Wash your genital area gently and frequently, using mild soap or no soap at all. Pat dry.
- If you suspect your vaginitis may be caused by irritation rather than an infection, avoid the suspected irritant for a time, or switch brands.
- Soak in a sitz bath—a bathtub containing six inches of warm water and ½ cup of vinegar—or douche twice a day with a cleansing douche using 2 tablespoons white vinegar diluted in one pint of warm water. Vinegar helps change the acid balance of the genital area and helps restore the normal population of organisms.
- Plain yogurt may help soothe irritated tissues and restore balance. Apply it directly to the outer tissues, or use a tampon dipped in yogurt and remove in one hour, or dissolve two tablespoons of yogurt in one pint of warm water and use as a douche.

- Cut out sweets from your diet during an infection and in general as a preventive measure.
- Other preventive measures, which may also speed healing, include: avoiding bubble baths, which can irritate delicate genital tissue; avoiding vaginal deodorants; minimizing clothing that encourages overgrowth of organisms by reducing air circulation, such as tight jeans, panty hose, and underwear made from synthetic fabrics; and spending as little time as possible in wet or damp clothing such as bathing suits or workout clothing.

Homeopathic Remedies

The most common homeopathic remedies for vaginitis are:

- Sepia. For a discharge that is yellow-green and smells offensive, and that is worse in the morning, from walking, and before a menstrual period. Accompanying symptoms are a feeling of pressure or heaviness in the pelvis, cramping, and burning pain and irritation of the vulva.
- Graphites. For a thin, nonodorous, white, burning discharge that often flows in gushes. Accompanying symptoms are weakness or abdominal tension. Symptoms are worse from walking and in the morning.
- Mercurius vivus. For a greenish, irritating discharge accompanied by rawness of the vulva; symptoms are often worse in the evening or at night; the vulva feels better after washing with cold water.

- Pulsatilla. For creamy white discharge; when the discharge is either bland or irritating. This remedy is especially useful for vaginitis that changes in character from day to day, and that occurs during pregnancy or in young girls.
- Calcarea carbonica. For thick white or yellow discharge that causes severe itching, may flow in gushes, and doesn't have much odor.

Dosage

Choose the remedy from the above list that most closely matches your symptoms. Administer following the Rule of Three (page 55). If the remedy does not prove to be effective, repeat the same process with the next homeopathic remedy that most closely corresponds with the symptoms.

Important Precautions

If you are presently taking allopathic drugs, or are under medical treatment for a specific medical condition, it is essential to consult your homeopath or allopathic doctor before administering homeopathic remedies. Medical care should also be sought if there is significant pelvic or lower abdominal pain; fever; you have had a recent new sexual partner and/or if you suspect you may have a sexually transmitted disease; the symptoms occur in a young (prepubescent) girl; there is a heavy discharge that does not improve with homeopathic self-care.

VOMITING

(See "Abdominal Pain and Indigestion.")

WARTS

Warts, also called "verruca," are skin growths related
to viruses. Common warts may crop up in the hands,
feet, and face; plantar warts are found on the soles of
the feet; and venereal warts affect the genitals and surrounding area. Wart viruses are contagious; however,
some people appear to be more susceptible than others.
Allopathy gets rid of the growths with caustic chemicals, electricity, freezing, and surgery. Homeopathy regards such measures as suppressive and potential
sources of deeper chronic disease.

General Homeopathic Home Care

- If you have only one or a few warts and they are
  not painful, the best course is to do nothing.
  With time, they usually go away by themselves.
- Sometimes hypnosis or the power of suggestion
  rouses the body's vital force to throw off the
  warts. Children can be encouraged to say
  "good-bye" to their warts as they stroke them
  two or three times every night before bed.

Homeopathic Remedies

Homeopathic remedies are very effective in treating
warts. The best remedy is a constitutional one, prescribed by an experienced professional. However, you

may want to try one of these remedies, commonly used
for acute conditions:

- Causticum. For warts anywhere on the body, especially the fingertips and face.
- Dulcamara. For large, smooth, flat warts on the
  back of the hand, on the fingers, or on the face.
- Antimonium crudum. For hardened smooth
  warts such as plantar warts.
- Thuja. For warts on the genitals, anus, or chin.
- Nitric acid. For warts on the genitals, anus, or
  lips; for soft, irregularly shaped warts; warts on
  stalks; painful or bleeding warts.

Dosage

Choose the remedy from the above list that most
closely matches your symptoms. Administer a single
dose. If the remedy does not prove to be effective, repeat the same process with the next homeopathic remedy that most closely corresponds with the symptoms.

Important Precautions

If you are presently taking allopathic drugs, or are under medical treatment for a specific medical condition,
it is essential to consult your homeopath or allopathic
doctor before administering homeopathic remedies.
Medical care should also be sought if the warts are on
the genitals; genital warts can be a sign of syphilis and
must be examined by a qualified medical professional.

FIRST AID FOR INJURIES

Injuries due to accidents and other causes are the easiest and most satisfying conditions to treat homeopathically, for several reasons:

- Compared with the conditions discussed in the previous section, injuries are relatively simple and straightforward problems. The injuries covered in this section are caused directly by an outside force; the effects are clear and immediate and the tissue changes are quite similar from person to person and even from mammalian species to species, especially during the first few days.
- There is simply less variety in the ways that people react to bites, burns, cuts, bruises, sprains and so on, than to colds, flu, menstruation, and bladder infections. Therefore, case taking is less complicated, and the number of remedies used is

considerably fewer than for other acute conditions.

• In treating injuries we match the particularly
  strong characteristics of a remedy with the common, dramatic symptoms that follow injury.
  Provings have shown that in a healthy individual, Arnica produces profound symptoms of
  bruised pains that are worse from touch and
  motion. On the other hand, Hypericum causes
  shooting nerve pain in healthy people. So it is
  easy to determine that Arnica is the most effective remedy immediately after a sprain, strain, or
  blunt trauma; and that Hypericum is the remedy
  for injuries to the nerves.

Allopathy treats injuries with drugs and techniques
that suppress inflammation and pain. Treating traumatic injuries homeopathically avoids suppressing
symptoms such as inflammation and pain. Rather, it
allows these natural healing mechanisms to do their
work. Inflammation, for example, removes disrupted
tissues and lays down the framework for tissues that
need to be rebuilt. Pain prevents us from using the injured part prematurely and disrupting the healing process. Homeopathy may allow us to feel a little more
pain than if we treat the injury allopathically, but a
little pain reminds us to listen to our body. Homeopathy relieves pain not by suppressing it, but by shortening healing time—the body doesn't require the pain
anymore as a healing tool. Sometimes dramatic relief
occurs after you have used a homeopathic remedy—but
remember, even if the pain disappears completely, you
have still been injured and need to rest because you

could slow the healing process if you do "too much too soon."

BITES

Bites and stings from insects, snakes, animals, or humans always result in some local reaction because of exposure to venom or saliva. This is the bodymind's way of preventing these substances (which may be harmful) from spreading to the rest of the body. Local reactions to most insect bites are not serious; however, systemic reactions occasionally occur and require emergency treatment. The main concern with animal bites (other than by pets) is the possibility of rabies.

General Homeopathic Home Care

- Pulling out an insect stinger may release more venom into the body; flicking it out with a fingernail or using a sterilized needle is a safer method of removal. Then bathe the sting or bite with cool water.
- If the bite is from a snake, seek immediate emergency medical attention and advice unless you are absolutely sure the snake is not poisonous. In this case, treat as you would a puncture wound (see page 264).
- Animal bites should be cleaned with soap and water and allowed to bleed as much as possible so any foreign material is flushed out and away. Then soak the bitten area in warm water several times a day for four days; this keeps the wound

open to allow bacteria and debris to drain so infection doesn't occur.

Homeopathic Remedies

The most common homeopathic remedies for bites are:

- Ledum. This is the most commonly used homeopathic remedy for insect and animal bites; use Ledum whenever there is redness, swelling, and stinging pain; when the area feels cold and feels better from applications of cold.
- Apis. For insect and animal bites that are red and swollen; when the area feels hot and feels worse with applications of heat. Apis is recommended as your second choice if Ledum has not brought improvement after four hours.
- Hypericum. The last remedy of choice; useful if there are sharp shooting pains. In addition to administering Hypericum orally, Hypericum tincture, diluted 10 drops per cup of sterile water, may be applied to the bite every half hour.

Dosage

Choose the remedy from the above list that most closely matches your symptoms. Administer following the Rule of Three (page 55). If the remedy does not prove to be effective, repeat the same process with the next homeopathic remedy that most closely corresponds with the symptoms.

Important Precautions

If you are presently taking allopathic drugs, or are under medical treatment for a specific medical condition, it is essential to consult your homeopath or allopathic doctor before administering homeopathic remedies. Medical care should also be sought if a bite turns very painful or itchy; the swelling worsens or spreads rapidly; the person has difficulty breathing; the sting is in the mouth or throat; the person has a history of allergic reaction to insect stings; the person feels faint or has difficulty breathing; there are signs of infection such as fever, pus, or extensive redness and swelling; a bite doesn't heal within two weeks; there is a possibility that the animal carries rabies; the bite is from a human; the bite is on the hand, or an animal bite is in the joint such as the knee; the bite may be from a poisonous snake.

BRUISES

Bruises are accumulations of blood under the skin, caused by the impact of a hard object. The blow breaks the blood vessels, allowing blood to leak out. The result is a "black-and-blue" mark and mild to severe pain, particularly when pressure is applied.

General Homeopathic Home Care

- Rest the injured part.
- Cover the injured area with a loose wrap to prevent further injury.

- Apply hot wet compresses or take a hot bath twelve hours after the injury to help healing.

Homeopathic Remedies

The most commonly used homeopathic remedies for bruises are:

- Arnica. This is the most often used remedy for bruises of any kind. Although Arnica is not a "painkiller," it speeds up healing to such a degree that the pain of the injury vanishes, sometimes miraculously. Arnica tincture or ointment may also be rubbed gently onto the area two to three times a day; or dilute 10 drops of tincture in $1/2$ to one cup of warm water and use as a wet dressing.
- Ledum. This is the remedy of choice for "black eyes," or when the bruise is severe and feels cold and numb, but feels better with application of cold. Ledum is also helpful if the bruise is very slow to heal.
- Ruta. For bruises and pain that affect bones like the shin, kneecap, or elbow.
- Conium. Use for injuries to the glandular tissue of the breast, after initially treating with Arnica.
- Bellis perennis. For injuries to the breast or testicle, after first using Arnica for two to three days. This remedy is also used for nerve injuries after first treating with Hypericum, especially when the pains are worse from a hot bath or a warm bed, and better from cool applications.
- Staphysagria. For testicle injuries that are still painful after Conium, or after two to three days

of Arnica when the testicle remains very painful from the slightest touch and is better from a warm bath or warm application.

Dosage

Choose the remedy from the above list that most closely matches your symptoms. Administer following the Rule of Three (page 55). If the remedy does not prove to be effective, repeat the same process with the next homeopathic remedy that most closely corresponds with the symptoms.

Important Precautions

If you are presently taking allopathic drugs, or are under medical treatment for a specific medical condition, it is essential to consult your homeopath or allopathic doctor before administering homeopathic remedies. Medical care should also be sought if the bruise is very severe and deep, and the affected area is very large; if you bruise easily and often; or if bruising occurs without obvious injury or is associated with bleeding elsewhere, such as the gums, nose, or rectum. Also seek medical care if the injury is to the breast or testicle.

BURNS

Burns may arise from many causes: from dry heat, such as fire, or from a hot object such as an iron or cooking tool; moist heat, such as steam or hot liquids; acids; or electricity. The least serious type of burn is a first-degree burn, such as most sunburns. The injury is superficial and the skin turns red and may be painful. A first-degree burn is usually treatable at home. Next comes the second-degree burn: deeper layers of the skin are affected and redness, pain, and blistering occur. Severe sunburns and scalding with hot water are common second-degree burns, and if not extensive can usually be treated at home as well. Third-degree burns are very serious, because all the skin layers are destroyed; the skin appears white or black and there is no pain because the nerve endings have been charred. Such burns cause fluid loss, infection, and scarring, and require professional emergency care.

General Homeopathic Home Care

- Apply cold water to the burn immediately and continue until the pain is gone (at least five minutes, and up to one hour). If possible, immerse the area in cold water or ice water; this stops further skin damage and eases pain. You may repeat the cold treatment if the pain returns.

- Avoid applying anesthetic cream or sprays, because this slows healing and may provoke an allergic reaction. Also avoid using butter, or nonhomeopathic creams or ointments.

- Avoid breaking any blisters that form, since they are nature's protective bandages. A bandage may shield the blisters from breakage or a burn from further injury, but otherwise covering the burn is not necessary.

- For chemical burns, read the label on the container for specific instructions; most recommend flushing the burn with water.

Homeopathic Remedies

The most common remedies for burns are:

Topical Remedies

- Calendula. Calendula lotion, or Calendula tincture (diluted 10 drops in ½ cup of sterile water) may be applied locally. In first-degree burns, apply every eight to twelve hours. In second-degree burns, apply every six to eight hours after blisters have burst. In third-degree burns, apply twice a day during the last stages of healing to reduce scarring.
- Hypericum. Hypericum tincture (diluted 10 drops in ½ cup of sterile water) may be applied to second-degree burns; apply gently so you don't break the blisters.

Internal Remedies

- Urtica urens. For first-degree or second-degree burns that are very painful.
- Cantharis. For second-degree or third-degree burns.
- Phosphorus. For electrical burns.

Dosage

Choose the remedy from the above list that most closely matches your condition. Apply topical remedies as indicated above; administer internal remedies following the Rule of Three (page 55). If the remedy does not prove to be effective, repeat the same process with the next homeopathic remedy that most closely corresponds with the symptoms.

Important Precautions

If you are presently taking allopathic drugs, or are under medical treatment for a specific medical condition, it is essential to consult your homeopath or allopathic doctor before administering homeopathic remedies. Medical care should also be sought if a second-degree burn is larger than the person's hand or involves the face or the hand; there is a third-degree burn of any size; there is an electrical burn or radiation burn; there is a chemical burn that is serious; there are signs of infection, such as fever, pus, extensive and increasing swelling or redness.

CUTS, SCRAPES, AND PUNCTURE WOUNDS

Cuts usually disturb only the skin and fatty tissue underneath and can be treated at home unless major blood vessels, tendons, or nerves have been severed or damaged. Scrapes are shallower and damage only the skin; even so, scrapes expose millions of nerve endings and so are usually more painful than cuts. Puncture wounds penetrate deep into the body tissues and may contain foreign material that is difficult to remove and increases risk of infection.

General Homeopathic Home Care

- If there is profuse bleeding from a cut, apply firm pressure directly on the cut, until the bleeding stops.
- Clean the cut or scrape with mild soap and warm water, making sure that no dirt, glass, or other foreign material is left in the wound.
- Wash a puncture wound with soap and water, removing as much foreign material as possible. Allow the wound to bleed as long as possible to encourage the flushing out of foreign material or germs. The exception is if the bleeding is severe or pulsating or squirting; in this case, apply pressure over the wound or, if the wound could contain a foreign body, press the nearest pressure point. (See a first-aid handbook for details.)
- Soak a puncture wound in warm water for fifteen minutes four times a day to keep the wound open and allow foreign material to be carried away.
- Cover the wound with a Band-Aid or gauze and tape (or wrap gently) to protect the wound and help absorb tissue fluids and debris.

Homeopathic Remedies

The most commonly used homeopathic remedies for cuts, scrapes, and puncture wounds are:

External Remedies

- Calendula. Apply this remedy to cuts or scrapes in either tincture form (diluted 10 drops in ½ cup sterile water); in lotion form; or, for scrapes only, in ointment or oil form. Apply two to four times a day, depending on the severity.

- Hypericum. When you have a cut that appears infected, apply the tincture (diluted 10 drops in ½ cup sterile water) directly to the wound, every hour for three hours and every three to four hours thereafter.

Internal Remedies

- Hypericum. If a cut is deep, painful, and sensitive to the touch, administer Hypericum orally in addition to applying it locally. Hypericum is also useful for cuts that affect nerve-rich parts of the body, such as the fingers or toes; for cuts that cause shooting pains; and for puncture wounds if there are sharp, shooting pains.
- Ledum. For all puncture wounds, especially when they are cold to the touch, but feel better with applications of cold.
- Apis. For puncture wounds that feel warm or hot, that sting with pain, and that improve with applications of cold.
- Arnica. For scrapes and cuts from blunt trauma that includes bruising.

Dosage

Choose the remedy from the above list that most closely matches your symptoms. Apply the external remedies as indicated. Administer internal remedies following the Rule of Three (page 55). If the remedy does not prove to be effective, repeat the same process with the next homeopathic remedy that most closely corresponds with the symptoms.

Important Precautions

If you are presently taking allopathic drugs, or are under medical treatment for a specific medical condition, it is essential to consult your homeopath or allopathic doctor before administering homeopathic remedies. Medical care should also be sought if there is profuse bleeding that direct pressure cannot stop; there is tingling or numbness near the injured part; there is a cut on the face, chest, abdomen, back, or palm; there is dirt or foreign matter that washing cannot remove; the edges of a cut cannot be kept together (because they may need stitches); there are signs of an infection such as fever, pus, extensive redness, and swelling; the person may need a tetanus shot; a puncture wound is very deep or is located anywhere except the limbs.

DENTAL TRAUMA

Many dentists prescribe homeopathic remedies to their patients to ease pain and avoid problems after traumatic dental procedures. You, too, can use homeopathic home care and remedies after you have had root canal or tooth extraction. Pain and inflammation surrounding the eruption of wisdom teeth also respond to homeopathy. Chronic toothaches also have many remedies, but require the care of a professional.

General Homeopathic Home Care

- Follow your dentist's instructions for rinsing and chewing and other postoperative care.

Homeopathic Remedies

The most common homeopathic remedies for dental trauma are:

- Arnica. For treating or preventing hemorrhaging (bleeding) after tooth extraction or dental surgery. Take twice a day for two days prior to dental work, as well as afterward.
- Hypericum. For pain after a tooth extraction or dental injection, especially if there is nerve tingling or shooting pains. Hypericum may be alternated with Arnica.
- Ruta. Take after initial treatment with Arnica for pain after dental surgery, especially if the bone was scraped or injured.
- Phosphorus. For bright red hemorrhaging after dental work.
- Lachesis. For dark red hemorrhaging after dental work.
- Belladonna. For throbbing pain around wisdom teeth.

Dosage

Choose the remedy from the above list that most closely matches your symptoms. Administer following the Rule of Three (page 55). If the remedy does not prove to be effective, repeat the same process with the

next homeopathic remedy that most closely corresponds with the symptoms.

Important Precautions

If you are presently taking allopathic drugs, or are under medical treatment for a specific medical condition, it is essential to consult your homeopath or allopathic doctor before administering homeopathic remedies. Medical care should also be sought if bleeding or pain persists despite treatment or if fever develops.

DISLOCATED JOINTS

Sometimes the force of a fall, a blow, or a strong yank pulls a bone out of its normal position in a joint. The most common dislocations involve the shoulder; however, knees, fingers, thumbs, elbows, hips, jaws, and ankles may dislocate as well. This is a serious injury with swelling, pain, discoloration, and a deformed appearance. Ligaments, tendons, nerves, and blood vessels may be involved and therefore the injury should be treated by a trained professional. Before and after professional treatment, homeopathic remedies can lessen pain and speed healing.

General Homeopathic Home Care

- Do not attempt to readjust the joint—leave that to a professional. Rather, immobilize the joint to protect it from further injury.

Homeopathic Remedies

The most common homeopathic remedies for dislocated joints are:

- Arnica. Administer Arnica immediately after the injury to minimize bleeding, shock, and pain, and to begin healing. Arnica may also be given if pain develops later on.
- Ruta. Administer after the joint has been relocated.
- Bryonia. If the dislocated joint becomes very swollen, and pain increases with the least little movement.

Dosage

Choose the remedy from the above list that most closely matches your symptoms. Administer following the Rule of Three (page 55). If the remedy does not prove to be effective, repeat the same process with the next homeopathic remedy that most closely corresponds with the symptoms.

Important Precautions

If you are presently taking allopathic drugs, or are under medical treatment for a specific medical condition, it is essential to consult your homeopath or allopathic doctor before administering homeopathic remedies. You should always seek medical care if you suspect a joint has been dislocated.

THE A-TO-Z GUIDE TO . . . TREATMENT

EYE INJURIES

Any type of eye injury should be taken seriously, because it could lead to loss or impairment of sight. Minor eye injuries that are treatable with home care include foreign objects in the eye such as dirt, sand, or dust; black eyes caused by a blow to the eye; and subconjunctival hemorrhage (leakage of blood from the blood vessels in the white of the eye), which usually occurs after a cough or sneeze, but sometimes for no discernible reason.

General Homeopathic Home Care

- If the problem is due to a foreign object, wash the eye with cool water to flush the irritant away. If this fails, roll or lift the eyelid and, with a cotton swab moistened with sterile water, try to gently remove the object.
- If the person has a black eye, use an ice pack initially (during the first twelve hours) and warm compresses thereafter.
- For a subconjunctival hemorrhage, apply a cool, wet cloth to the closed eye.

Homeopathic Remedies

The most commonly used homeopathic remedies for eye injuries are:

- Calendula, Hypericum, or Euphrasia. For a *foreign object* in the eye, use any one of these tinctures (diluted 10 drops in 1 cup sterile water) as an eyewash to soothe the eye after the object has been removed. Use Calendula if the eye is simply irritated and painful, Hypericum if the pain is sharp, and Euphrasia if the pain is associated with profuse tearing.

- Arnica. Use for a *black eye* to relieve the pain and heal damaged tissues; most useful when the pain is worse from damp cold. Use Arnica for a *subconjunctival hemorrhage* to relieve pain and reabsorb the blood.
- Ledum. Use after initial treatment with Arnica for a *black eye* or *subconjunctival hemorrhage* to help the blood reabsorb and return the tissues to a normal color.
- Symphytum. Use after initial treatment with Arnica if there is pain in the eye after blunt trauma.
- Hamamelis. For *subconjunctival hemorrhage* if Arnica doesn't work, or if the blood returns after Arnica has helped the body reabsorb it.

Dosage

Choose the remedy from the above list that most closely matches your symptoms. Administer following the Rule of Three (page 55). If the remedy does not prove to be effective, repeat the same process with the next homeopathic remedy that most closely corresponds with the symptoms.

Important Precautions

If you are presently taking allopathic drugs, or are under medical treatment for a specific medical condition, it is essential to consult your homeopath or allopathic doctor before administering homeopathic remedies.

Medical care should also be sought if you have any question about the seriousness of an eye injury; if the cornea is involved in any way; or if you cannot remove a foreign object from the eye or if something is embedded in the surface of the eye. Seek immediate evaluation if there is a change of vision, if the cornea becomes cloudy or shows blood beneath it, or if a foreign body has punctured the eye.

FRACTURES

Though the injury may be painful, it isn't always obvious when a bone is broken or fractured. Fractures often mimic sprains (see "Sprains and Strains") because of the swelling; however, the pain is usually confined to a smaller area than in a sprain. Another clue is when the bone appears misshapen, which occurs in certain types of fractures. Any bone in the body can break when a strong force—usually caused by a fall—puts more stress on the bone than it can withstand. Most fractures heal in four to twelve weeks, depending on your age and severity of injury. A broken bone needs professional treatment to set (realign) it correctly; some fractures require surgery. However, homeopathy can help the body repair and replace the damaged bone. If the person may be in shock, see "Shock."

General Homeopathic Home Care

- Do not press on a suspected fracture or attempt to realign the bone, since this may injure the tissue further. Do not attempt to move or put weight on the injury. You may wrap gently the most common fractures that occur around the home—those of the finger, wrist, or foot; this helps immobilize the area to minimize pain and further damage while the person is transported to a medical professional.

Homeopathic Remedies

The most common homeopathic remedies for fractures are:

- Arnica. This is the remedy to give immediately after a bone has been injured or broken. It eases pain and swelling, and helps prevent the person from going into shock.
- Ruta. Useful if the pain of the injury is worse when beginning to move, but better from gentle, continuous motion.
- Symphytum. After the injury has gotten professional care, administer Symphytum to continue the healing process and "knit" the bone tissue back together; when the pain of the fracture is worse from use and motion.
- Bryonia. This is sometimes used specifically for broken ribs.
- Silica. This remedy is useful when the bone has been "chipped"—tiny pieces have broken off, as in a severe ankle sprain.

Dosage

Choose the remedy from the above list that most closely matches your symptoms. For most broken bones, administer Arnica for five days; then once the pain and swelling have healed, administer Symphytum in a low potency (3 or 6c) twice a day for up to three weeks. If the remedy does not prove to be effective, or if there are special indications for Ruta, Bryonia, or Silica, repeat the same process with the next homeopathic remedy that most closely corresponds with the symptoms.

Important Precautions

Consult a physician *immediately* anytime you suspect a fracture. Seek medical care if the injury is serious; the back, neck, thigh, or pelvis may have been broken; the person is in shock; or the injured limb is numb, cold, has a bluish tinge, or is not usable. Get medical attention also if the pain or swelling and discoloration worsen or if the ability to use the part decreases over time.

HEAD INJURIES

Active children are particularly prone to head injuries, but we can bump our heads at any age. Fortunately, most head injuries are not serious. Although such bruises may result in "goose eggs" (a swelling in the skull and scalp), the brain itself is well cushioned and protected from injury. The size of the bump is not a reliable indication of the seriousness of the injury; to determine, you need to watch the person carefully at home (or in a hospital).

General Homeopathic Home Care

Home care consists of observing the person for a few days after a bad injury has occurred. A minor injury to a child after a fall (for instance, off a chair or out of a tree) may stun the child temporarily, but he does not lose consciousness. The child may cry, and may vomit once or twice during the first hour or two; but this, too, is mild and soon subsides. After a minor injury, the child is usually his old self within eight hours. Symptoms caused by more severe head injuries indicate that you should get medical care (see "Important Precautions" below).

Homeopathic Remedies

The most common homeopathic remedies for a head injury are:

- Arnica. This remedy is called for when the pain from a head injury is worse from movement and pressure, and better from rest; the mental dullness following a trauma to the head is a good indicator for Arnica.
- Hypericum. Use this remedy if the symptoms of pain include buzzing, tingling, or other nervelike sensations.

Dosage

Choose the remedy from the above list that most closely matches your symptoms. Administer following the Rule of Three (page 55).

Important Precautions

If you are presently taking allopathic drugs, or are under medical treatment for a specific medical condition, it is essential to consult your homeopath or allopathic doctor before administering homeopathic remedies. Medical care should also be sought if you notice any of the following; they are signs of a severe head injury and usually take several hours or even days to develop: lethargy, confusion, loss of memory, slurred speech, or unconsciousness; pupils of unequal size, or blurred or double vision; severe vomiting that persists and gets worse; a seizure or convulsion; severe or persistent headache; blood from an ear or the nostrils; slow or irregular breathing or pulse. All falls in the elderly should be examined for hidden fractures. In addition, you should seek professional care if the above symptoms appear and worsen slowly; this may indicate that blood is accumulating inside the skull, which eventually puts dangerous pressure on the brain. (This condition is rare, but more common in the elderly, because they fall frequently and because many are on medication that hampers blood clotting.)

HEAT EXHAUSTION OR HEATSTROKE (SUNSTROKE)

Our bodies vary in their ability to handle the extra heat generated by hard work or play, especially if we are in a hot, humid, or poorly ventilated environment. Signs of overheating, heat exhaustion, or heat stress are dizziness, fainting, or giddiness; excessive sweating; cold, moist, pale skin; thirst; extreme weakness or fatigue;

headache; nausea and vomiting; muscle cramps; and a rapid, weak pulse. Left untreated, heat exhaustion can progress to heatstroke; symptoms include loss of consciousness; confusion; red, hot skin; and a fast pulse. Heatstroke can lead to permanent brain damage or death and requires emergency medical treatment.

General Homeopathic Home Care

- Move to a cool or shady area to rest.
- Drink water or other fluids; some advise salt tablets, salted water (½ tsp salt in 8 ounces of water), or a "sports drink" such as Gatorade.
- Apply warm, moist compresses to cramping muscles, followed by gentle massage.
- Apply cool compresses to forehead, neck, and armpits to help cool the blood; fanning will also help bring down body temperature and is especially important when the person has heatstroke.

Homeopathic Remedies

The most common homeopathic remedies for heat exhaustion or heatstroke are:

- Veratrum album. This is the most often used remedy for all the symptoms of heat exhaustion.
- Cuprum metallicum. When symptoms of heat exhaustion include severe muscle cramps, muscle twitches, and convulsions.
- Belladonna. For treatment of heatstroke while awaiting medical treatment.

THE A-TO-Z GUIDE TO . . . TREATMENT

Dosage

Choose the remedy from the above list that most closely matches your symptoms. Administer following the Rule of Three (page 55). If the remedy does not prove to be effective, repeat the same process with the next homeopathic remedy that most closely corresponds with the symptoms.

Important Precautions

If you are presently taking allopathic drugs, or are under medical treatment for a specific medical condition, it is essential to consult your homeopath or allopathic doctor before administering homeopathic remedies. Medical care should also be sought if there are signs of heatstroke, such as unconsciousness or rapid pulse; if symptoms of heat exhaustion do not improve within one hour, or become more severe.

NOSEBLEEDS

Nosebleeds are usually due either to injury to the blood vessels inside the nose, such as from nose picking or vigorous blowing; or to irritation from a virus, such as a cold virus or other irritants such as pollen or smog. They may also occur as a result of change in air pressure, such as happens during airplane travel. The occasional nosebleed is not serious and can be handled at home. Recurrent or severe nosebleeds should be investigated by a medical professional.

General Homeopathic Home Care

- To stop bleeding, sit down and squeeze the nose between thumb and forefinger just below the hard, bony cartilage. Applying pressure for five minutes or so usually is sufficient.
- Do not stuff the nose with gauze or tissue.
- If the bleeding is associated with a cold virus, or the dry, heated air common in winter, treat the cold (see "Colds"), and humidify the indoor air.

Homeopathic Remedies

The most commonly used homeopathic remedies for nosebleeds are:

- Arnica. When the cause is an injury.
- Phosphorus. For mild nosebleeds with bright red blood that just won't stop oozing.
- Ferrum metallicum. For nosebleeds in children.
- Lachesis. For nosebleeds that are due to blowing the nose, especially if the blood is dark red.
- Kali bichromicum. When the blood is dark red and is accompanied by a dry stuffiness, tension, and tingling high up in the nose.

Dosage

Choose the remedy from the above list that most closely matches your symptoms. Administer following the Rule of Three (page 55). If the remedy does not prove to be effective, repeat the same process with the next homeopathic remedy that most closely corresponds with the symptoms.

Important Precautions

If you are presently taking allopathic drugs, or are under medical treatment for a specific medical condition, it is essential to consult your homeopath or allopathic doctor before administering homeopathic remedies. Medical care should also be sought if the person has frequent nosebleeds; the reason for the nosebleed cannot be identified; the bleeding is profuse and lasts more than thirty minutes; the bleeding is mild and lasts more than three hours.

SHOCK

After any kind of serious injury, the person is in danger of going into shock. Shock may also follow a severe allergic reaction (anaphylactic), an infection, or choking. Shock occurs when not enough blood flows through the body, putting vital organs at risk of permanent damage, and which may result in death. The symptoms are: pale or "ashen" skin; perspiration; dilated (wide-open) pupils; the person also appears to be lethargic, acts "shocky," or loses consciousness, takes shallow or irregular breaths, and has a weak pulse or heart rate. Shock is a medical emergency and requires immediate professional care; in the meantime, homeopathy can help minimize and reverse the symptoms.

General Homeopathic Home Care

- Keep the person warm, by covering with blankets if necessary. Have her lie down with feet slightly elevated to encourage blood flow to the head; do not bend the knees.

- Do not move the person if she is seriously injured.
- The person may drink small sips of water if she wishes.

Homeopathic Remedies

The most common homeopathic remedies for shock are:

- Arnica. This is the most often indicated remedy for shock and should be given immediately.
- Aconite. If the symptoms of shock are accompanied by restlessness and fear.

Dosage

While waiting for professional help, choose the remedy from the above list that most closely matches your symptoms. Administer following the Rule of Three (page 55). If the person is unconscious, you can safely place the pellets under the tongue, on the tongue, or inside the cheek while awaiting emergency care.

Important Precautions

If you are presently taking allopathic drugs, or are under medical treatment for a specific medical condition, it is essential to consult your homeopath or allopathic doctor before administering homeopathic remedies. Always seek medical care if you suspect the person is in shock or is going into shock.

SMASHED FINGERS AND TOES

Fingertips and toes often get into trouble—caught in drawers and doors, under hammers or other people's feet. The smashed tissues throb and discolor from leaking blood vessels, and minor bone fractures may accompany the soft-tissue damage. The finger or toe swells and is painful; the nail may tear or eventually fall off but grows back in four to six weeks. Though painful and inconvenient, smashed fingers or toes are usually treatable at home.

General Homeopathic Home Care

- Do not remove a bashed or torn nail; you should clip off the nail only if it is loose or is likely to catch on other objects.
- Immobilize the injured digit with a thick gauze wrap and/or tape it to the adjacent digit, making sure that the wrap doesn't prevent the free flow of blood and tissue fluid.
- If blood under a fingernail is causing pressure and pain, see your doctor or go to an emergency room.

Homeopathic Remedies

The most common homeopathic remedies for smashed fingers and toes are:

- Hypericum. This is the standard remedy for injuries to areas that are richly supplied with nerves, including fingers and toes.

- Arnica. Use this remedy if Hypericum doesn't help.
- Ledum. Useful during the second stage of healing, after Hypericum or Arnica has been administered for two to four days; especially recommended if the skin or nail is broken or the bruising and swelling are not decreasing easily.
- Hypericum or Calendula tincture may be used as a wet dressing or soak. Dilute 10 drops of tincture in ½ to 1 cup of water; apply for fifteen minutes, two to three times a day.

Dosage

Choose the remedy from the above list that most closely matches your symptoms. Administer following the Rule of Three (page 55). If the remedy does not prove to be effective, repeat the same process with the next homeopathic remedy that most closely corresponds with the symptoms.

Important Precautions

If you are presently taking allopathic drugs, or are under medical treatment for a specific medical condition, it is essential to consult your homeopath or allopathic doctor before administering homeopathic remedies. Medical care should also be sought if the end of the finger or toe is deformed, or if the part turns red, swollen, or drains pus, or if a fracture or other severe trauma is suspected.

SPLINTERS

When tiny shards of wood or glass become embedded in the skin, pain and infection can result. Homeopathic treatment encourages the body to expel or wall off the foreign body.

General Homeopathic Home Care

- Clean the affected area with soap and water and soak in warm water for fifteen minutes twice a day.
- Use a heat-sterilized needle and/or tweezers to remove a splinter embedded near the skin surface.
- Keep the area covered with a sterile bandage, but do not use any skin healers such as Calendula so the wound will not be stimulated to close prematurely.

Homeopathic Remedies

The most common homeopathic remedies for splinters are:

- Ledum. Use initially for the pain and swelling.
- Silica. Use in a low potency (3–6c) during the second stage of healing to help expel the foreign body.

Dosage

Begin treatment with Ledum, following the Rule of Three (page 55). When symptoms subside, use Silica three times a day.

Important Precautions

If you are presently taking allopathic drugs, or are under medical treatment for a specific medical condition, it is essential to consult your homeopath or allopathic doctor before administering homeopathic remedies. Medical care should also be sought if you cannot remove the splinter; or if the area shows symptoms of infection such as redness, swelling, or pus.

STRAINS, SPRAINS, AND MUSCLE INJURIES

Ligaments are the tough, fibrous bands of tissue that connect the bones of a joint to one another to keep them stable yet mobile. Tendons are the tissues that attach muscles to bones. The system works fine during most of our daily activities, but sports, rough or normal play, and falls and other mishaps occasionally take their toll. Under conditions of overuse or strong force, either or both forms of connective tissue can be overstretched, resulting in a *strain;* or they may be partially torn, resulting in a *sprain.* (Complete tears are rare.)

The symptoms of a strain are immediate and continuing pain and slow swelling; a sprain or complete tear tends to be painful but swells more quickly and becomes discolored from the blood leaking out of damaged blood vessels. The most commonly injured joints are the wrist, ankle, knee, and shoulder, and of course the elbow, as in the infamous "tennis elbow." Sprains and strains generally take four to six weeks to heal, and home care and homeopathy can ease the process.

When we injure a muscle, the tiny fibers that make up the "meat" of the muscle are torn. The more fibers that tear, the more severe the muscle injury. Any muscle can be hurt, but large muscles in the back (see "Back and Neck Problems"), chest, thigh, bicep, or calf are most often affected. Muscles are injured by overwork or overstretching, usually while lifting a heavy object, a sudden strain during a fall or playing sports, or doing something we are unaccustomed to, such as shoveling snow or being a "weekend athlete." The symptoms of pain and stiffness, which may be immediate or delayed by several hours, are more quickly and effectively healed with the help of homeopathy.

General Homeopathic Home Care

- Rest the injured area and exercise caution in your activities to avoid injuring the tissue further. Do not move the area if it hurts; you may find crutches, splints, and slings help support and immobilize the joint and aid healing.
- Elevate the affected area, but do not apply ice or cold compresses, because this prevents nature's splint from fully forming and helping to heal the injury.
- Wrap the injured part firmly, but not too stiffly, with an elastic bandage.
- After the first twenty-four hours, apply wet heat (use a hot water bottle or heating pad with a

moist cloth placed over the skin) for fifteen minutes two to three times a day. After twenty-four
to forty-eight hours, soaking the area in a hot
tub may also speed healing.
- As healing progresses, begin to use the area
slowly and gently to restore mobility and flexi-
bility.
- Avoid using allopathic products for injuries;
these usually contain strong-smelling substances
such as camphor and can interfere with the effectiveness of homeopathic remedies.

Homeopathic Remedies

The most common homeopathic remedies for strains,
sprains, and muscle injuries are:

- Arnica. This is the most strongly indicated remedy for immediate treatment of severe pain,
swelling, and inflammation from these injuries.
It is usually used for two to four days when the
injury is worse from any motion or exertion. Arnica oil or tincture, applied twice a day locally,
also eases pain. You may use both oral and topical forms when pain is severe.
- Rhus toxicodendron. Use after initially treating
with Arnica; for all moderate strains, sprains,
and muscle injuries when pain and stiffness are
worse during initial motion and improve with
continued motion.
- Bryonia. For sprains and strains that feel worse
during both initial motion and during continued
motion.
- Ruta. Administer after the initial swelling, pain,

and inflammation subside, or if Rhus toxicodendron has not helped healing, or if the injury is
not affected one way or the other by motion.
This is the remedy of choice for "tennis elbow"
and other conditions when the injury occurs at
the point of attachment to the bone.
- Ledum. Most effective for ankle injuries, especially when the injured area feels numb or cold,
and improves when cold is applied.

Dosage

Choose the remedy from the above list that most
closely matches your symptoms. Administer following
the Rule of Three (page 55). If the remedy does not
prove to be effective, repeat the same process with the
next homeopathic remedy that most closely corresponds with the symptoms.

Important Precautions

If you are presently taking allopathic drugs, or are under medical treatment for a specific medical condition,
it is essential to consult your homeopath or allopathic
doctor before administering homeopathic remedies.
Medical care should also be sought if a joint seems too
loose, cannot be straightened, or is misshapen; there is
severe pain or swelling; there is intense muscle spasm;
the affected limb is distorted; the affected area is cold,
numb, or has a bluish tinge; the joint or limb can't be
used or bear weight within twelve hours or if this is still
quite difficult after seventy-two hours; the person is
weak, pale, faint and sweaty; or if symptoms fail to
improve despite homeopathic treatment. Also consult a

professional if it is possible that a bone has been fractured (particularly likely if a child has fallen on an outstretched hand); such injuries often involve a wrist fracture, which is difficult to detect.

PART III

. . . .

A Glossary of Homeopathic Remedies

There are nearly three thousand single homeopathic remedies, with two to three hundred in common use. This section includes the remedies appropriate for self-treatment that are most often listed in Part II, "The A-to-Z Guide to Common Conditions," in this book. The glossary provides you with more detailed information about the individual remedies in order to help you more closely match the person's total symptom picture —the physical, emotional, and mental state.

ACONITE (MONKSHOOD) AK-o-night

Aconite is made from an herb. Hahnemann proved the remedy in 1805, and it soon became the homeopathic replacement for bloodletting, which had been the primary treatment for fever and inflammation. A fast-acting medicine, Aconite is most useful at the very first signs of an acute condition that comes on suddenly and with intensity. Complaints appear soon after exposure to cold, dry air, from the intense heat of summer, or after some kind of shock. The symptoms are characterized by inflammation, redness, dryness, and anxiety. The pain is often stinging, burning, cutting, or stabbing; the person may scream with pain and be inconsolable. Aconite is often used for colds, dry coughs, sudden fevers, headache, injuries accompanied by fear and restlessness, measles, burning sore throat, palpitations, and acute rheumatism. People who benefit from Aconite are generally vigorous; they may have a hot, red face and look anxious or nervous; they are usually thirsty for cold drinks.

Symptoms are worse: in a warm room; in the evening and at night; from lying on the affected side; from music or noise, touching, and tobacco smoke; from exposure to dry, cold wind.

Symptoms are better: in the open air; after sweating; with rest.

ALLIUM CEPA (RED ONION)   AL-ee-um SEE-pah

As anyone who has ever sliced an onion knows, Allium causes our eyes to tear and our nose to run. Therefore, homeopathically prepared Allium is used to treat conditions that produce these same symptoms: colds, allergies, eye inflammations, headaches, sneezing, and sore throat. This remedy is indicated when the discharge from the nose is watery and irritating, and the watery tears from the eyes are bland.

Symptoms are worse: in a warm, stuffy room; in the evening; from sitting.

Symptoms are better: in fresh air; in a cold room; from motion.

AMBROSIA

(See "Allergies: Hay Fever.")

ANTIMONIUM TARTARICUM
(ANTIMONY) An-ti-MOAN-ee-um tar-TAR-i-kum

Antimonium is derived from a mineral that many years ago was used to cause vomiting. Antimonium is therefore useful for digestive symptoms (especially in children); it is also used for chest infection (in both children and the elderly) characterized by loud coughing with great rattling of mucus, but little expectoration. The person who needs Antimonium is usually thirstless, pale, and sweaty, and has a white coated tongue. Children tend to be irritable, but do not want to be touched. Adults tend toward despondency, anxiety, and apathy.

Symptoms are worse: from cold, damp weather; from lying down at night; from getting angry; in a warm room.

Symptoms are better: from belching, vomiting, bringing up phlegm, sitting erect, being in motion, and lying on the right side.

APIS MELLIFICA (HONEYBEE)
AY-piss mel-i-FIGH-ka

Apis is prepared from the sting of the honeybee, and the symptoms for which it is useful are similar to those of a bee sting. These include sharp, stinging pains, rosy redness, and swelling; they occur with a rapid, violent intensity. The symptoms are either right sided or begin on the right and move toward the left. People who require Apis are apathetic, fearful, irritable, jealous, restless; they are whiny, clumsy, and uncoordinated; they are not thirsty. Apis is especially useful for bites, urethritis, skin infections, sore throats, eye infections, hives, and fever.

Symptoms are worse: with touching; in a warm room or with heat; in late afternoon; on the right side; after sleeping.

Symptoms are better: in the open air; with applications of cold water; after uncovering.

ARNICA MONTANA (WOLFSBANE)
AR-ni-kah mon-TAN-ah

Made from a perennial herb, Arnica is best known for its ability to promote healing, control bleeding, reduce swelling, reduce shock, and promote blood reabsorption due to injuries. It is best administered immediately after almost any trauma including bruises, black eyes, sprains and strains, fractures. Arnica is indicated if the person is thirsty, if the pain feels sore and bruised, if he doesn't want to be moved. Another key symptom is that of restlessness and the feeling that everything he lies on feels too hard.

Symptoms are worse: from light touch or jarring movement; from exposure to heat; from lying on the injured part.

Symptoms are better: from lying down with the head low.

ARSENICUM ALBUM (WHITE ARSENIC)
Ar-SEN-i-kum AL-bum

Arsenicum is prepared from the mineral arsenic, which in crude amounts is a deadly poison. This remedy is commonly used to treat diarrhea, food poisoning, and other digestive problems; headaches; colds, sore throats, asthma, and coughs; fever; cystitis and insomnia. Anxiety, restlessness, burning pain, chills, and thirst are important characteristics; the hours around midnight are common times of crisis. People who benefit from Arsenicum catch cold easily; they are chilly, pale, meticulous, and afraid they have a serious or deadly illness; they feel weak and exhausted, often out of proportion to their illness.

Symptoms are worse: from exposure to cold, drafts, and dampness; with cold food and drinks; at night; with exertion.

Symptoms are better: with heat, hot drinks, and a warm bed; from lying down.

BELLADONNA (DEADLY NIGHTSHADE)
bel-ah-DON-ah

The Belladonna remedy is made from a flowering plant that has long been used as an herbal remedy. In homeopathy it is used to treat parts of the body that have become inflamed or infected, that turn red, radiate heat, and throb painfully. Common conditions include fever, headache, earache, menstrual cramps, skin infections, colds, flu, and sore throat (before there is any color to the mucus). The person who needs Belladonna has a face that is red and flushed, the eyes sparkle or shine and the pupils are dilated, and the fever is high and results in hot perspiration, delirium, and/or twitching muscles. Symptoms that respond to Belladonna come on suddenly and intensely, worsen rapidly, and subside quickly.

Symptoms are worse: from bright light, cold air, touch, noise, and jarring movement.

Symptoms are better: from rest and lying down, particularly on the abdomen; from bending the head backward; from darkness and quiet.

BORAX

(See "Thrush.")

BRYONIA ALBA (WILD HOPS)
bry-OH-nee-ah AL-bah

Bryonia comes from a vine that grows wild in England and Europe; only the root is used for homeopathy. It is used principally for complaints that worsen (often dramatically) from any kind of motion, even deep breathing or moving the eyes. This remedy acts slowly but deeply, for problems that come on slowly. These include headache, fever, flu, dry cough (with pain on coughing), laryngitis (when hoarseness is worse from talking), sharp joint and muscle pain, respiratory problems, and digestive problems. People who benefit from Bryonia are slow and sluggish mentally and physically; when ill they are irritable and want to be still and left alone. They may have dry skin, lips, and mucous membranes, are usually thirsty for large sips, and prefer cold liquids.

Symptoms are worse: from any motion; from heat; in warm rooms; in the summer; at 9:00 P.M.

Symptoms are better: in cool open air; from applications of cold or warmth; from application of pressure and lying on the painful side; while lying down.

CALCAREA CARBONICA (CALCIUM CARBONATE)   kal-CA-ree-ah kar-BONN-i-ka

This is a form of calcium obtained from the middle layer of oyster shells. Individuals who fit the Calcarea symptom picture are usually pale, plump, flabby; lack mental and physical endurance; sweat easily (often a single body part) yet have trouble keeping warm; she may crave eggs or undigestible things such as chalk. Calcarea is often used for slow-healing injuries; for conditions that appear after exposure to cold or wetness, and include sore throat, colds, and bronchitis; and at the end of a cold for lingering symptoms of morning cough, nasal odor, and sinus pain.

Symptoms are worse: with mental or physical exertion; from exposure to cold; from moist air or wet weather; during a full moon.

Symptoms are better: from dry, warm air and weather; from lying on the painful side.

CALCARICA SULPHURICA

(See "Acne.")

CALENDULA (MARIGOLD)   ka-LEN-du-lah

The homeopathic remedy is made from the juice of the leaves, blossoms, and buds of the plant. Calendula is a good, all-around remedy for all kinds of skin problems, wounds, and cuts—applied externally as an ointment, tincture, or as an internal remedy. There are no strong mental or emotional components of the total symptom picture; nor are there any marked modalities that make the symptoms better or worse.

CANTHARIS   kan-THAR-uss

This remedy is made from an alcohol extract of a handsome green beetle known as the Spanish fly. Contrary to common belief, it is not a true aphrodisiac. Cantharis is a powerful urinary and skin irritant that, when prepared homeopathically, is used to treat acute inflammations such as bladder infections, "honeymoon cystitis" (a common urinary irritation in women that occurs after sex), urethritis, and burns.

Symptoms are worse (bladder problems): from cold drinks; before, during, and after urination.

Symptoms are better (burns): from cold compresses.

CAUSTICUM

(See "Bedwetting.")

CHAMOMILLA (CHAMOMILE)   kam-oh-MEEL-ah

Chamomilla is a plant that has long been used as an herbal remedy. Homeopathically it is suitable for people who are irritable, discontented, and inconsolable; for children who are prone to screaming tantrums; and for people who hate to be touched and are extremely sensitive to pain. Complaints often are related to teething, anger, or too much coffee or tea; and are accompanied by sweating and sometimes a high fever. Chamomilla is commonly used for ear pain, especially when symptoms are eased by wrapping the ear warmly and when the child is carried.

Symptoms are worse: during the evening; from fresh air, wind, and cold; from anger; from heat, or touch.

Symptoms are better: from being carried and rocked.

CISTUS CANADENSIS

(See "Mononucleosis.")

COFFEA (Coffee)

(See "Insomnia.")

COLOCYNTHIS   kol-o-SIN-this

Colocynthis is made from bitter cucumber and is used for severely painful conditions, such as menstrual cramps, headache, sciatica, or digestive cramps. People who require this remedy liken their agonizing abdominal pains to being squeezed between two stones; the pain forces them to double over.

Symptoms are worse: from eating fruit (abdominal pains); from touch (headache); on the right side (sciatica).

Symptoms are better: they are relieved by hard pressure (neuralgic pains and cramps).

DULCAMARA

(See "Allergies: Hives.")

EUPHRASIA (EYEBRIGHT)   you-FRAY-ja

Prepared from a small flowering plant, this homeopathic remedy is used to treat eye problems related to many conditions, such as hay fever and colds. Any kind of eye discharge may be helped by Euphrasia, including those that are bland or irritating, thin and watery, or thick and sticky. People with hay fever benefit from this remedy if they have a profuse and irritating eye discharge and a bland nasal discharge. There are no strong mental or emotional components of the total symptom picture.

Symptoms are worse: in the evening; indoors; from warmth; from south winds; from light.

Symptoms are better: in the dark; from coffee.

FERRUM PHOSPHORICUM (PHOSPHATE OF IRON) FER-um foss-FOR-i-kum

Most often used during the early stages of conditions characterized by inflammation, such as earache, colds, cough, and fever. Ferrum phosphoricum shares many symptoms with Aconite and Belladonna, except that the symptoms may not come on as rapidly. The person who needs Ferrum phosphoricum typically is nervous, sensitive, and pale, with fever-flushed cheeks, has a throbbing headache, is sensitive to cold, and easily exhausted.

Symptoms are worse: at night; between 4:00 and 6:00 A.M.; from motion, touching, or jarring.

Symptoms are better: from applications of cold.

GELSEMIUM (YELLOW JASMINE) jel-SEE-mee-um

The homeopathic remedy is prepared from the roots of this flowering plant and is best suited to people who are mentally and physically dull and sluggish; they feel drowsy and have heavy limbs and eyelids that droop closed. Gelsemium is often prescribed for fright (such as stagefright when the person's mind goes blank and becomes dull), anxiety, flu, and migraine headache. It is used for fever when it comes on over a few days, especially when accompanied by creeping chills up and down the back.

Symptoms are worse: from damp weather; from fog; before a storm; from bad news; from anxiety surrounding an anticipated event.

Symptoms are better: with sweating; after urination; in open air.

GRAPHITES   gra-FIGHT-ees

Graphites is made from fine English pencil lead, which is a combination of carbon and iron. It is used for timid, fidgety, nervous, indolent people who are chilly, catch colds, are overweight, and often constipated. Their skin often looks unhealthy; every injury gets infected, and eruptions ooze a sticky, honeylike liquid.

Symptoms are worse: at night; from warmth; from getting chilled.

Symptoms are better: in the dark; from being wrapped up.

HEPAR SULPHURICUM (CALCIUM SULPHIDE)   HEE-par sul-FERR-i-kum

This is a form of calcium prepared from oyster shells and sulphur and is used homeopathically for people who feel chilly, hate the cold, and catch colds easily. Their colds and other conditions are characterized by puslike discharges that often smell like cheese. People who need Hepar tend to be angry, impulsive, irritable, and do things quickly. They are very sensitive to all impressions, including pain (which tends to be sharp and splinterlike), pressure, and verbal insults. Hepar is useful in treating conditions that include skin infections, laryngitis, boils, and inflammations of the ears, eyes, throat, and skin.

Symptoms are worse: from cold drinks and cold air;

from the slightest draft; from movement; from touch; from lying on the painful side.

Symptoms are better: from damp weather; from wrapping up the body, especially the head; from exposure to heat; after eating.

HYPERICUM PERFOLIATUM (SAINT-JOHN'S-WORT) High-PERR-i-kum per-fol-ee-AY-tum

The remedy made from this herb is helpful in healing injuries that involve the nerves, such as back injuries after a fall, or injuries to fingers and toes, as well as bites, burns, cuts, and dental trauma. The tincture is valuable in skin and ear problems. The person feels pains that are shooting (especially along nerves), burning or tingling, severe, and sensitive to touch or pressure.

Symptoms are worse: from exposure to cold; from pressure.

Symptoms are better: from bending the head back.

IGNATIA IMARA (SAINT IGNATIUS BEAN) ig-NAY-she-ah ih-MA-rah

This remedy is prepared from the bean of a shrub that was named by the Jesuits. People who fit its symptom picture are sensitive, delicate, moody, conscientious, idealistic, and introspective. They do not express their feelings openly, but may sigh deeply. Ignatia is useful for symptoms that follow severe emotional upset such as grief, shock, anger, disappointment, or embarrassment. People who need this remedy may have head-

ache, insomnia, or contradictory symptoms such as a
lump in the throat or sore throat that feels better when
swallowing, or nausea that is relieved by eating.

Symptoms are worse: in the morning; from open air;
after eating; with exposure to tobacco or coffee or external warmth.

Symptoms are better: while having a good time; exposure to heat; while eating; from changing positions.

IPECAC (IPECACUANHA OR BRAZIL ROOT)   i-pe-KAK

Ipecac is prepared from the root of a shrub that grows
in Central and South America. Most people are familiar
with Ipecac in its herbal form, which is used to cause
vomiting in case of poisoning through ingestion. When
prepared homeopathically, this remedy is mostly used
for digestive problems; it is also useful for asthma if
nausea accompanies the breathing problem. People
who require Ipecac have violent and persistent symptoms; they look pale, break out in a cold sweat, and are
sensitive to cold and to warmth.

Symptoms are worse: in the morning; from a moist,
warm wind; in winter and dry weather.

Symptoms are better: in the open air.

KALI BICHROMICUM (BICHROMATE OF POTASH)   KAY-ligh bi-KROH-mi-kum

Prepared from a potassium compound, this remedy is
used for sinus problems, headache, colds, sore throat. It
is particularly useful when these conditions produce a

thick, sticky, yellow or greenish mucous discharge that
is difficult to expectorate or blow out, a crust in the
nose, and small pains that move around or come and
go and are characteristically sharp. This remedy is typically used for sinus problems when there is thick mucus
and pain at the root of the nose that is better from
warm, wet compresses. The symptom picture includes
listlessness, irritability, indifference, a sensitivity to cold
and drafts, and the tendency to get cold easily.

Symptoms are worse: between 2:00 and 3:00 A.M.
and upon awakening; from lying on the affected part;
from cold, damp weather; from being uncovered.

Symptoms are better: from heat; in the open air;
from eating; during hot weather.

LACHESIS (SNAKE VENOM)   LAK-e-siss

A remedy derived from the venom of the South American bushmaster snake, Lachesis is often prescribed to
treat symptoms of menopause, such as hot flashes, or
hormonal headaches; sore throats also respond to this
remedy, as do spring hay fever, nosebleeds, and ulcers.
People whom this remedy helps are tired and are not
rejuvenated after sleeping; their breath may smell; and
their symptoms often occur on the left side and then
may move to the right. They are anxious and sluggish
when they awaken in the morning, but are generally
talkative, restless, exhilarated, and "volcanic" by nature. Symptoms are often related to overwork or personal loss.

Symptoms are worse: with heat; in the morning;
when wearing tight clothes; before a menstrual period;
from drinking alcohol; with humidity.

Symptoms are better: in fresh air; while eating; after a menstrual period (or any discharge) starts.

LYCOPODIUM (CLUB MOSS)
ligh-ko-POH-dee-um

Lycopodium is prepared from the pollen of a trailing evergreen plant; this remedy has been found in the medicine pouches of ancient European cave dwellers. It is useful for a variety of conditions, including earaches, sore throats, digestive problems, skin rashes, and cystitis; symptoms characteristically are worse on the right side or move from right to left. The indigestion, distension, and gas are worsened by beans, cabbage, and starches. This remedy benefits people who crave sweets, prefer warm drinks, and like fresh air; they tend to be insecure and even cowardly, uneasy in social situations, filled with self-doubt but intolerant of contradiction, headstrong, and haughty.

Symptoms are worse: between 4:00 and 8:00 P.M.; in a hot room; after sleeping; when wearing tight clothing.

Symptoms are better: with movement; in cool air; with warm food and drinks; after midnight.

MAGNESIA PHOSPHORICA (MAGNESIUM PHOSPHORUS)   mag NEE-jah fos-FOR-i-kah

When homeopathically prepared, this mineral salt relieves cramping pains such as menstrual cramps, abdominal pain with nausea and vomiting, neuralgic pain, and teething pain. There are no strong emotional or mental symptoms for this remedy.

Symptoms are worse: from the cold; from touch; from being uncovered; from fresh air.

Symptoms are better: from heat; from firm pressure; from bending over double.

MERCURIUS (MERCURY) mer-KYU-ree-us

This homeopathic remedy is prepared from either of two forms of the metal mercury: Mercurius vivus and Mercurius solubilis; they are used interchangeably for the same symptoms. Mercury is indicated for a variety of conditions that are characterized by pus formation and inflammation, such as ear and eye infections, sore throat, cystitis, and skin infections. Generally, individuals who need this remedy have foul-smelling breath, perspiration, urine, and phlegm; they sweat profusely, tend to have mouth problems, and their teeth leave an impression around the edge of their soft tongue. Like a mercury thermometer, they are extremely sensitive to extremes in temperature. Their nights are restless and sweaty, but the sweat does not make them feel better. They are intensely thirsty for cold drinks.

Symptoms are worse: from hot or cold; during the evening or at night; from lying down on the right side; in the open air; after eating sweets; from moving around.

Symptoms are better: from moderate temperature.

NATRUM MURIATICUM (SODIUM CHLORIDE; TABLE SALT)   NAY-trum myur-ee-AT-i-kum

As one would expect, the conditions treated by this remedy made from common salt tend to involve a disturbed water balance. People needing Natrum muriaticum are extremely thirsty, have eczema or acne, and dry skin and lips (which may be cracked); they sweat profusely when ill and all their body discharges are thin and watery. They are sad, but hold in their feelings, cannot cry in public, and are aggravated by consolation. They tend to be constipated and have difficulty urinating in the presence of other people. Symptoms often appear after an emotional trauma such as loss, rejection, or a reprimand. Headaches, hay fever, and insomnia are common complaints that respond to this remedy.

Symptoms are worse: between 10:00 and 11:00 A.M.; with exposure to sun or heat; after eating; before a menstrual period; with noise or music; at the seashore.

Symptoms are better: with open air; cold bathing; after lying down; from fasting or skipping meals; with pressure against the back.

NUX VOMICA (SEEDS OF THE POISON-NUT TREE)   nux VOM-i-kah

Nux vomica is prepared from the powdered seeds of an evergreen tree. It is used to treat a wide variety of symptoms, many of which relate to digestive conditions (such as nausea, vomiting, constipation, and hemorrhoids) and problems resulting from an overindulgence in alcohol, coffee, and allopathic medications (such as hangovers, headaches, and sleeplessness). People needing Nux vomica are quick, nervous, and irritable; they tend to be workaholics and suffer from mental stress. Noise, odors, light, touch, and interruption are intolerable. They feel chilly and catch colds easily. Spasms, cramps, asthma, and neuralgic pains are influenced by Nux vomica.

Symptoms are worse: after eating; in the morning; from mental exertion; from spicy food, coffee, alcohol, tobacco, and other stimulants; from loss of sleep; from the cold.

Symptoms are better: with heat; after uninterrupted naps; from lying or sitting down; from hot drinks.

PETROLEUM

(See "Allergies: Eczema" and "Motion Sickness.")

PHOSPHORUS   FOSS-for-us

This remedy is made from white phosphorus, a form of this element that is highly flammable and burns with a white flame. Those who need Phosphorus tend to be pale, tall, and slender; they are always hungry because of their speedy metabolisms. They are very thirsty for cold drinks, but feel chilly and dislike the cold. They bleed easily and have burning pains. Such individuals are weak and delicate; they have little stamina and are prone to exhaustion. Yet they are very quick, animated, artistic, extroverted, and crave company. They are very susceptible to external impressions such as light, odors, touch, and thunderstorms. Phosphorus is used most often for coughs, respiratory problems, hoarseness, sore throat, ear problems, and nosebleeds.

Symptoms are worse: in the evening; during thunderstorms; when lying on the left side; from weather changes; from the cold.

Symptoms are better: after sleeping; from cold drinks; from massage; in the open air; from lying on the right side.

PULSATILLA (WINDFLOWER) pul-sa-TIL-ah

Pulsatilla is prepared from a flowering plant and has been called the queen of homeopathic remedies because it is so widely used, especially in women. People who benefit from Pulsatilla have dry mouths and lips, but are not thirsty. Their body discharges are thick, and yellow or green. They may have rheumatic aches and pains that frequently change locations. They dislike fatty foods, which cause digestive problems. These individuals have mild, gentle, affectionate, moody, and weepily sensitive and changeable dispositions; children tend to be clingy and need attention especially when sick. They dislike heat and prefer fresh, open air, and sometimes cold weather. Pulsatilla is often given for chicken pox, colds, coughs, digestive problems, eye and ear infections, and menstrual problems.

Symptoms are worse: from exposure to heat; after rich or hot food and drinks; from wet weather or wind; in the evening; from a warm room.

Symptoms are better: in the open air; from gentle motion; after cold food and drinks; from cold applications.

RHUS TOXICODENDRON (POISON IVY)
russ tox-i-ko-DEN-dron

The remedy prepared from this poisonous plant mainly affects the skin and mucous membranes, and the joints, tendons, and ligaments. People who require Rhus toxicodendron are generally chilly, hate the cold and damp, and feel as if the coldness is running through their veins. They feel achy, sore, or tearing needlelike pains, and their joints may be stiff or swollen. Symptoms may begin after exertion or overexertion. They are restless mentally and physically, and can't stay comfortable in any one position for long. They may feel despondent and fearful; be unquenchably thirsty; and have a red-tipped tongue. This remedy is often used for flu, chicken pox, mumps, herpes, poison ivy, or poison oak.

Symptoms are worse: from the cold and damp; at night; during rest, initial movement, and prolonged movement.

Symptoms are better: from warmth and dryness; from motion; from change of position or continued gentle movement; from sweating; from pressure on sore spots; while lying on a hard surface.

SABADILLA

(See "Allergies: Hay Fever.")

SEPIA (CUTTLEFISH) SEE-pee-ah

Sepia is prepared from the ink of the cuttlefish, a sea creature related to the octopus and squid. The remedy is often prescribed for symptoms relating to menstrual disorders and menopause, for hemorrhoids, constipation, sinus infections, and headaches. People needing Sepia are pale and sallow and have circles under the eyes; they are chilly and sensitive to the cold. They feel exhausted and run-down; they are indifferent and apathetic, and can be moody. They crave sour, spicy foods and chocolate, and feel an emptiness emotionally and in the stomach, which food fails to satisfy. Women who benefit from Sepia may feel a bearing-down sensation in the pelvic area and sadness before or during the menstrual period.

Symptoms are worse: between 4:00 and 6:00 A.M.; in the evening; around the time of the menstrual period; from emotional upset; from exposure to cold.

Symptoms are better: after eating; after strenuous exercise; after running, fast walking, or dancing; with heat, pressure, or drawing the limbs up.

SILICA (FLINT) SIL-i-kah

Silica is a mineral remedy that best suits people who are very sensitive to cold and have icy cold hands and feet; they catch cold easily, and the symptoms often settle in the throat and are prolonged. They are nervous, confused, shy, conscientious, irritable, and sensitive to noise and pain. They cannot tolerate alcohol and are disgusted by meat. People who need Silica lack stamina and are easily worn out. Because of their sluggish metabolism, many of the conditions for which Silica is used relate to poor assimilation and sluggish digestion, such as weakness, headache, and constipation; Silica is also useful for coughs that linger after a cold.

Symptoms are worse: from cold, damp, and drafts; from bathing; from being uncovered; from cold food or drinks; from being consoled.

Symptoms are better: from exposure to heat; being dressed warmly; from wrapping the head.

SPONGIA TOSTA (SEA SPONGE)
SPON-jee-ah TOS-tah

This homeopathic remedy is made from a sponge that has first been toasted. Spongia is effective for treating coughs, colds, laryngitis, and breathing problems such as asthma. Individuals who need Spongia wake up with a feeling that they are suffocating and cannot wear tight clothing because of the problems with breathing.

Symptoms are worse: after sleep; from exposure to cold wind; from motion; from tobacco.

Symptoms are better: from lying with the head low.

SULPHUR (BRIMSTONE)   SUL-ferr

This homeopathic remedy is prepared from the fine yellow-greenish powder that is widely found in nature and around volcanoes. Homeopathic Sulphur is used in people who flush and are sensitive to heat, have red faces and lips and hot feet. They are thirsty, sweat profusely, and their body discharges are usually hot, foul smelling, and burning. They are lean and hungry, and must eat frequently and don't gain weight. They stoop and slouch, and are selfish, messy, and dirty. Symptoms that call for Sulphur include itching, burning, and pus-producing skin conditions; burning pains; acne; diarrhea; and fever.

Symptoms are worse: from warmth; from a warm bed; from standing; from washing; at 11:00 A.M.; from rest; at night; from alcohol.

Symptoms are better: in the open air; from warm drinks; from motion.

TABACUM (TOBACCO)

(See "Motion Sickness.")

TELLURIUM

(See "Ringworm.")

URTICA URENS (STINGING NETTLE)
UR-ti-kah YUR-ins

The homeopathic remedy prepared from this common plant has a few uses in acute skin conditions, including contact dermatitis, scalds, sunburn, hives, and herpes when the pain itches, stings, and burns. It also is used to antidote the ill effects of eating shellfish. There are no marked general symptoms.

Symptoms are worse: from touch; from water; from cool, moist air.

Symptoms are better: none.

VERATRUM ALBUM

(See "Diarrhea.")

WYETHA

(See "Allergies: Hay Fever.")

Appendix: Resources

HOMEOPATHIC ORGANIZATIONS

National Center for Homeopathy (NCH)
801 N. Fairfax Street, Suite 306
Alexandria, VA 22314
703-548-7790
  Serves as a clearinghouse for homeopathic information.
Sponsors yearly summer courses for health professionals or
lay people. Holds annual conferences. Sells books and litera-
ture as well as audio- and videotapes, publishes a monthly
newsletter and directory of licensed practitioners of homeopathy in the United States and Canada, and sponsors a network
of homeopathic study groups.

American Institute of Homeopathy (AIH)
1585 Glencoe St., #44
Denver, CO 80220
  The oldest national medical organization in the United
States and the main association of homeopathic medical doc-
tors. Holds annual meetings and publishes a journal.

International Foundation for Homeopathy (IFH)
2366 Eastlake Avenue E., Suite 329
Seattle, WA 98102
206-324-8230

Focuses on "classical homeopathy." Publishes a magazine and provides a training program for licensed professionals. Has a homeopathic referral service and a directory of IFH-trained practitioners. Teaches an advanced acute homeopathy course open to lay people. Publishes an annual book of cases cured by homeopathy.

Hahnemann Medical Clinic
828 San Pablo Avenue
Albany, CA 94706
510-524-3117

The largest homeopathic clinic in the United States. Has formed the Hahnemann College of Homeopathy, which provides a two-year training program for licensed professionals, considered to be one of the most rigorous in the country.

National College of Naturopathic Medicine
11231 SE Market Street
Box RES
Portland, OR 97216
503-255-4860
John Bastyr University of Naturopathic Medicine
144 NE 54th Street
Seattle, WA 98105
206-523-9585

Both of these four-year full-time colleges offer extensive training in homeopathy as part of their naturopathic medical training, and graduate courses as well.

MAIL ORDER SUPPLIERS

Homeopathic remedies are available in a growing number of health food stores and pharmacies. If you cannot locate a local supplier for the remedies you need, the following companies will send individual remedies to you by mail; many also supply homeopathic remedy kits and books on homeopathy.

Boericke and Tafel, Inc.
2381 Circadian Way
Santa Rosa, CA 95407
800-876-9505

Boiron, USA
6 Campus Boulevard, Building A
Newtown Square, PA 19073
800-BLU-TUBE

Dolisos America, Inc.
3014 Rigel Avenue
Las Vegas, NV 89102
800-365-4767

Hahnemann Medical Clinic
828 San Pablo Avenue
Albany, CA 94706
510-524-3117

Homeopathic Educational Services
2124 Kittredge Street
Berkeley, CA 94704
510-649-0294; 800-359-9051

Standard Homeopathic Company
210 W. 131st Street
Box 61067
Los Angeles, CA 90061
800-624-9659

Washington Homeopathic Products
4914 Del Ray Avenue
Bethesda, MD 20814
800-336-1695

Further Reading

Blackie, Margery. *The Patient, Not the Cure: The Challenge of Homeopathy*. Santa Barbara: Woodbridge Press Publishing Co., 1978.

Castro, Miranda. *The Complete Homeopathy Handbook*. New York: St. Martin's Press, Inc., 1990.

Coulter, Harris. *Homeopathic Science and Modern Medicine: The Physics of Healing with Microdoses*. Berkeley: North Atlantic Books, 1981.

Cummings, Stephen, and Dana Ullman. *Everybody's Guide to Homeopathic Medicines: Taking Care of Yourself and Your Family with Safe and Effective Remedies*. Los Angeles: Jeremy P. Tarcher, Inc., 1991.

Subotnick, Steven. *Sports and Exercise Injuries: Conventional, Homeopathic, and Alternative Treatments*. Berkeley: North Atlantic Books, 1991.

Ullman, Dana. *Discovering Homeopathy* (previously titled *Homeopathy: Medicine for the 21st Century*). Berkeley: North Atlantic Books, 1988.

Vithoulkas, George. *The Science of Homeopathy*. New York: Grove Press, 1980.

————. *Homeopathy: Medicine of the New Man.* New York: Arco, 1979.

Weiner, Michael, and Kathleen Gross. *The Complete Book of Homeopathy.* New York: Bantam Books, Inc., 1981.

Wood, Robert. *Homeopathy: Medicine That Works!* Pollock Pines, CA: Condor Books, 1990.

Index